Henry Gray

Henry Gray
1870–1938
Surgeon of the Great War

TOM SCOTLAND and ANN BOYER

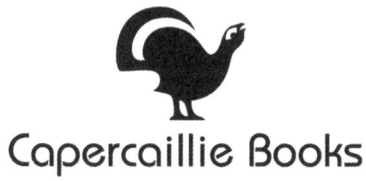
Capercaillie Books

First published by Capercaillie Books Limited in 2015.
Registered Office Summit House, 4–5 Mitchell Street, Edinburgh EH6 7BD

© Tom Scotland apart from Chapters 2 and 7 where © Ann Boyer

The moral rights of the authors have been asserted.

A catalogue record of this book is available from the British Library

ISBN 9781909305373

This book is sold subject to the condition that it shall not by way of trade or otherwise, be lent, resold, hired out or otherwise circulated without the publisher's prior consent in any form of binding or cover other than that in which it is published and without a similar condition including this condition being imposed on the subsequent purchaser. All rights reserved. No part of this publication may be reproduced, stored in a retrieval system or transmitted in any form or by any means, electronic, mechanical or otherwise without the written permission of the publisher.

Printed by Bell and Bain Ltd, Glasgow

This book is dedicated to

ALEXANDER ADAM, FRCS
1920–2009

*who always did his best to ensure that Aberdeen
medical graduates received due recognition.*

EVA ESTHER GRAY IVENS
1885–1968

*In loving memory of my grandmother,
whose lifelong faith in her brother Henry has inspired
my contribution to this book.*

Contents

Family Tree	8
List of figures	11
Acknowledgements	13
Preface	15
Foreword	17
Introduction	19
Chapter 1 Henry Gray Surgeon of the Great War	23
Chapter 2 Gray's family background	27
Chapter 3 Gray's career before the Great War	56
Chapter 4 Gray's career during the Great War	79
Chapter 5 Gray's career after the Great War	112
Chapter 6 An appraisal of Gray's surgical career	138
Chapter 7 Gray's closing years and death	154
Appendix I Gray's publications	159
Bibliography	165
Index	169

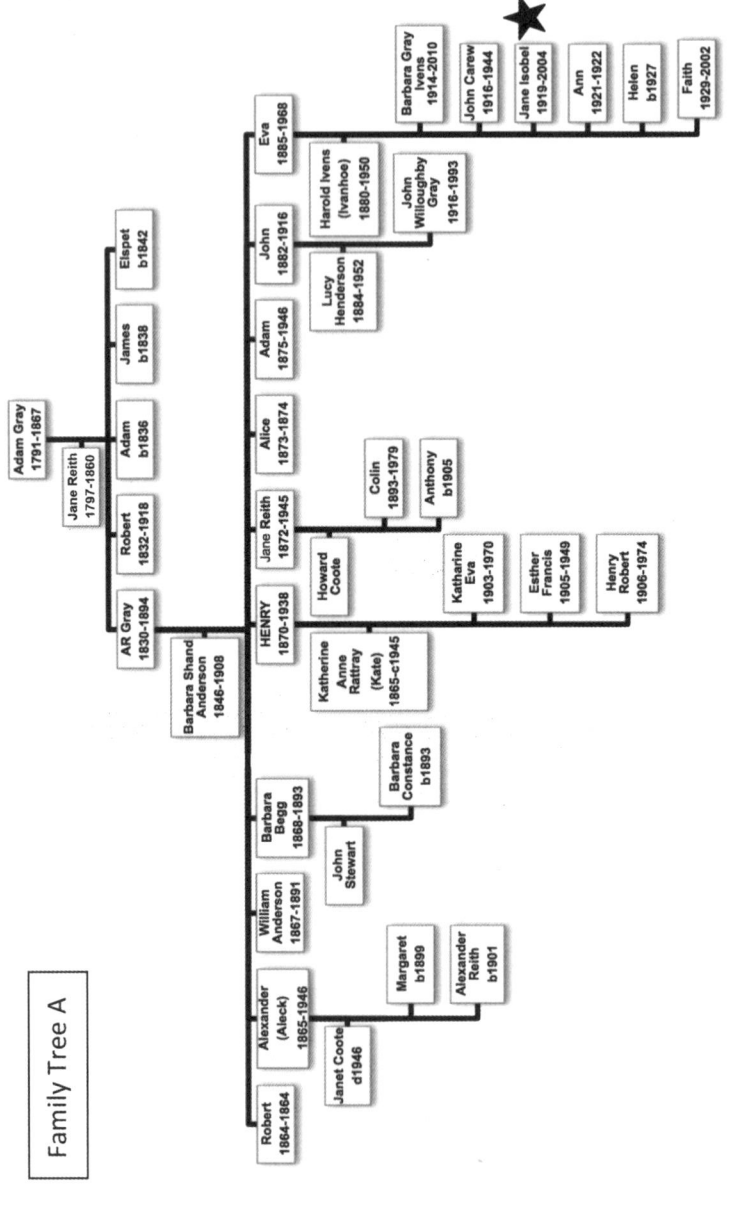

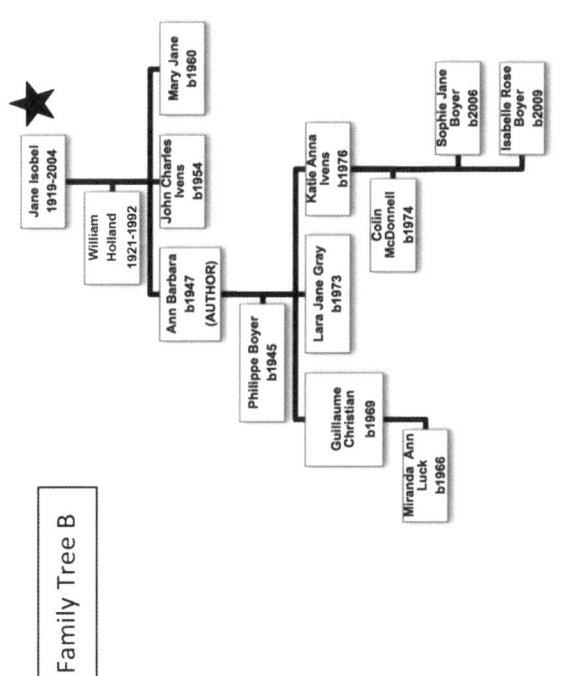

List of Figures

Figure 2.1	Alexander Reith Gray, c 1888 Author's own collection	25
Figure 2.2	Eva Esther Gray in 1890 aged five Author's own collection	30
Figure 2.3	Merchiston Castle 1st XV, 1888, Merchiston Castle School, Edinburgh Courtesy of Merchiston Castle School. Henry Gray is centre front	34
Figure 2.4	Eva and John Gray: c 1905 Author's own collection	39
Figure 2.5	Henry Gray taking delivery of a new car with Katharine and Esther at the back in bonnets, c 1907 Author's own collection	47
Figure 3.1	Marischal College, part of University of Aberdeen Author's own collection	53
Figure 3.2	Portrait of Sir Alexander Ogston Courtesy of Aberdeen Medico-Chirurgical Society	53
Figure 3.3	Sir Alexander Ogston at surgery illustrating antiseptic surgery; Ogston is on far left of the photograph. There is a carbolic dispenser on the far right to spray the wound and instruments with carbolic acid. Courtesy of Aberdeen Medico-Chirurgical Society	55
Figure 3.4	Henry Gray as a young man Author's own collection	60
Figure 3.5	Old Aberdeen Royal Infirmary at Woolmanhill Author's own collection	63
Figure 3.6	Cartoon of Henry Gray Courtesy of Aberdeen Medico-Chirurgical Society	65
Figure 3.7	Sir Berkeley Moynihan Author's own collection	66

Figure 3.8	Sir Robert Jones Author's own collection	67
Figure 3.9	Moynihan Club, Henry Gray 2nd row far left; Sir Berkeley Moynihan, centre front row; Robert Jones, front row far right Courtesy Professor James Hutchison, Regius Professor of Surgery, University of Aberdeen and Moynihan Chirurgical Club	68
Figure 3.10	Gray's home 34 Albyn Place, Aberdeen Author's own collection	73
Figure 3.11	Gray in photograph Aberdeenshire Cricket Club; Gray front row, far right Courtesy Mr Howard Smith and Aberdeenshire Cricket Club	73
Figure 4.1	Evacuation pathway for the wounded Courtesy Gordon Stables, Dept of Medical Illustration, University of Aberdeen	75
Figure 4.2	Soldiers in Oldmill Hospital (1st Scottish General Hospital) mending deep sea fishing nets in the restorative workshop Courtesy Aberdeen Medico-Chirurgical Society	87
Figure 4.3	Fractured femur. This is a high energy injury and there are four separate parts to the fracture Author's own collection	90
Figure 4.4	Rifle Splint Royal Army Medical Corps Training Handbook. London: HMSO, 1911, p. 345	90
Figure 4.5	Thomas Splint Author's own collection	91
Figures 4.6(a) and (b)	Extracts from Henry Gray's letter to his sister Eva	105
Figure 5.1	Henry Gray in later life Courtesy Dr Ian Levack	109

Acknowledgements

The authors are very grateful to Professor Kingsley Falconer, Past President of the Royal Australasian College of Surgeons, for writing the foreword, and to Dr Robert Galway for providing the preface. They are also grateful to Colonel Mike Stewart, RAMC (retd.) for his review of the work.

They wish to thank the Headmaster at Merchiston Castle School and Amy McGoldrick, Club Secretary, The Merchistonian Club, Merchiston Castle School, for providing the photograph of the school rugby team (Figure 2.3) and the information relating to Henry Gray's schooling in Chapter 2. They wish to acknowledge the Aberdeen Medico-Chirurgical Society for Figures 3.2, 3.3, 3.6 and 4.2 and Professor Jimmy Hutchison, Regius Professor of Surgery, University of Aberdeen and the Moynihan Chirurgical Club for Figure 3.9. They are very grateful to Mr Howard Smith and the Aberdeenshire Cricket Club for Figure 3.11., Mr Gordon Stables, Department of Medical Illustration, University of Aberdeen, for Figure 4.1 and Dr Ian Levack for Figure 5.1. Despite extensive and careful searches, it was not possible to find copyright ownership of Figures 3.7 and 3.8., which have been designated as Author's own collection. If copyright ownership subsequently comes to light then the orthopaedic co-author apologises and will give an undertaking to give appropriate acknowledge should there be any subsequent printings of this work.

The authors would like to thank Mr Colin Johnston, who provided helpful information about various locations in Aberdeen relevant to this biography and for his constructive comments after he read the draft chapters. They would also like to thank Mr Ken Mills for his personal memories of the wearing of surgical gloves at the Westminster Hospital in London in the 1950s. They wish to acknowledge their spouses, Lyn and Philippe, for their help, patience and understanding while the work to restore Henry Gray's name was undertaken.

Tom Scotland would like to thank Mr Christopher Lyons, head librarian of the Osler Library, Montreal, for helping with his enquiries and is grateful to Theresa Rowat, Director and University Archivist, McGill University Archives, for much painstaking work undertaken on his behalf to provide the relevant pages from Sir Arthur Currie's diary and associated correspondence relating to Sir Henry Gray.

Ann Boyer would like to thank her aunt, Helen Leach (nee Ivens) and niece of Henry Gray, for her interest in this project and her assistance in retracing family history.

Finally, she would like to pay tribute to her aunt, Barbara Gray Ivens, eldest daughter of Eva Esther Gray Ivens and niece of Henry Gray, for preserving, sorting and documenting the Gray family archives before her death in 2010 aged 95. Her dedication and hard work made a significant contribution to the enrichment of this biography.

Preface

The scholarly and principled work by Scotland and Boyer 'Henry Gray – Surgeon of the Great War' is a 'fine' but challenging read. It is challenging, given the immensity of detail and the background information presented. The accolade 'fine' is earned in its brevity as the authors clearly make their case for the redemption of Gray's long blighted reputation. Canadians have long tipped their hats to Aberdeen granite,[1] but have to date withheld a nod of approval in the direction of Sir Henry Gray.

In the words of Woodrow Wilson, Presidential politics sharpens the wit, but University politics dulls the sword. Even Sir Arthur Currie exited this saga with his weapon dulled.

One adjunct lesson stands out from this publication and that is the creative power that arises from the union of curiosity with serendipity.

A final observation to offer is the coincidental timing of publication of this treatise on Henry Gray with the permanent closure, earlier this summer, of the Royal Victoria Hospital which dates its beginning to 1893.

Robert Galway, BA, MD, FRCS(C)
Orthopaedic Surgeon (retd.) Toronto, Canada

---

[1] Stonemasons from Aberdeen, who had extensive experience working with granite, played a major role in the construction of the Rideau Canal between Kingston and Ottawa. Work began in 1827 and was completed in 1832. The exquisite stonemasonry is admired to this day.

Foreword

This well researched and engagingly written biography on Sir Henry Gray describes a robust, resourceful, complex, courageous and industrious Aberdonian surgeon of great integrity and innovative flair whose contributions towards the logistical and clinical management of the wounds sustained on the Western Front in the Great War were outstanding and remain historically important.

He recognised that the surgical management of modern high impact battlefield wounds amongst soiled fields resulting in gross tissue damage and contamination was often inadequate and led to many preventable deaths due to hypovolaemia and sepsis. His major long lasting innovation was that of introducing and then publicising (in June 1915, the same month that the Australian surgeon, Edward Milligan independently published) thorough debridement and wide local excision of non-viable tissue in a systematic fashion, principles which saved thousands of lives during that war and many more since. Those principles remain valid today.

He also appreciated the phenomenon of haemorrhagic shock and the need for adequate fluid replacement, the additional hazards of hypothermia, the crucial role of adequately splinting compound fractured femurs in particular and the importance of early definitive care of wounded patients.

His military surgery skills and achievements, and the high esteem with which he was held by his surgical colleagues in France and Flanders, are well recorded and have been fully recognised by official Australian and New Zealand military historians. Some limitations in the skills of diplomacy and eloquence meant that his achievements were not always as well appreciated back in Britain, in London or even in Aberdeen.

The travails of the war, along with personal losses during it, took their toll. His resumption of surgical practice in Aberdeen was characterised by fatigue and some loss of a sense of purpose.

The opportunity for a change came when an invitation to become Surgeon-in-Chief was sent by Sir Henry Vincent Meredith, President of the Royal Victoria Hospital of Montreal, with the unauthorised assumption that it would be combined with the role of Professor of Surgery, a teaching and research role for which he was not well suited, within the Department of Surgery of McGill University, Montreal.

That assumption was incorrect and Henry Gray became the main casualty in the subsequent battle over the joint appointments eventually leading to humiliation and having neither. His subsequent career was spent in relative surgical obscurity in Montreal until his death.

The biography emphasises and honours the permanent contributions which Henry Gray has made to surgery and to the ongoing care of the wounded. It also addresses the importance of taking great care and providing absolute clarity when offering and accepting significant appointments in surgery, and indeed in all walks of life.

Professor Kingsley Faulkner AM, MBBS (UWA), FRACS
School of Medicine, Fremantle
University of Notre Dame Australia
Past President, Royal Australasian College of Surgeons.

Introduction

Tom Scotland

The name of Aberdonian surgeon Sir Henry Gray (1870–1938) was first drawn to my attention by one of my predecessors in the orthopaedic department of Aberdeen Royal Infirmary, the late Professor Alexander Adam, a most distinguished and knowledgeable surgeon who became the librarian of the Aberdeen Medico-Chirurgical Society when he retired in 1983. Alex held this position right up until his death on 20 December 2009. He came across Henry Gray's name in the library in 2008 and found a couple of articles which suggested he had been a noteworthy surgeon, particularly during the Great War. Knowing of my interest in the history of that conflict, Alex gave the information to me and it soon became clear that Gray was responsible for many important pioneering surgical procedures between 1914 and 1918 and was subsequently knighted for his work as well as being awarded an Honorary LLD by the University of Aberdeen. Despite his many achievements, his name is scarcely known in his home city today. I also read some very uncomplimentary remarks about Gray in an article published in 2003 in the Canadian Bulletin of Medical History entitled *The Principal and the Dean*, which revealed that his previously distinguished career suffered a major reversal in Montreal after he had been appointed Surgeon-in-Chief to the Royal Victoria Hospital in 1923. Following a series of events which subsequently became known as 'The Sir Henry Gray Affair' and which culminated in his virtual dismissal from this position, he ended his working life in surgical obscurity. It seemed to me that Gray's fall from grace was not his fault but was due to bitter political infighting between Sir Henry Vincent Meredith, President of the Royal Victoria Hospital and Sir Arthur Currie, Principal and Vice-chancellor of McGill University, over the issue of whether Gray should be offered the Chair of Surgery at McGill. Since discovering this injustice I have made efforts to redress the balance and restore Gray's name to somewhere near its rightful place by writing papers for peer reviewed journals and by delivering lectures. I decided some years ago that I should write his biography and as the evidence for his surgical prowess during the Great War grew ever stronger, so did the need to write this book. I am very grateful to Dr Richard Cruess, co-author of *McGill Medicine*, (published in 2006) who suggested to me that a only a full scale biography would provide an opportunity for me to attempt to rehabilitate Henry Gray's name in the eyes of McGill University. This is certainly too much to expect since the present day perception of Gray in Montreal is based entirely on existing documentation in the McGill Archives which is invariably uncomplimentary. Perhaps a more realistic goal would be to gain an acceptance that Gray made major contributions to war surgery and if not *the* best was certainly *one of the best* 'hands on' military surgeons working in France during the Great War. Given the unfortunate end to his previously distinguished surgical career, it might also be conceded that some of the less than complimentary remarks made about him during his time at the Royal Victoria Hospital were unjustified.

Having decided then to write a biography, there was a major stumbling block because I was unable to find any of Gray's descendents and I had no access to important background family information. Then on 25 October 2012, I delivered a lecture at the National Army Museum in London entitled 'War Surgery 1914–18.' A video was made of the lecture which soon found its way onto *youTube*. This caused considerable amusement amongst my former colleagues, since I had always been regarded as a complete dinosaur in matters relating to information technology. On 5 June 2014, a lady by the name of Ann Boyer happened to find the video on the National Army Museum website. She watched it and posted the following comment.

Introduction

Sir Henry Gray was my great uncle. He was my maternal grandmother's elder brother and she nursed with him in Aberdeen before the First World War. He dedicated a copy of *The Early Treatment of War Wounds*[1] to her, which is now in my possession. I'm researching family history in my retirement and would like to thank Mr Scotland for his account of WW1 British orthopaedic surgery (which I have only just tumbled upon!).

When I read Ann's comment, my first thought was one of relief that she had thought my talk was worth listening to. I also realised that I must make contact with her, which I very promptly did, since this was too good an opportunity to miss. The rest, one could say, is history, and Ann and I have now combined forces to write the biography of this great Aberdonian surgeon.

---

1 Gray, H.M.W., *The Early Treatment of War Wounds*. London: Henry Frowde and Hodder & Stoughton, 1919.

CHAPTER 1

Henry Gray (1870–1938)

Surgeon of the Great War

'Cometh the hour, cometh the man'

This biography sets out to show that Henry Gray (1870–1938) was one of the most skilful and innovative surgeons to serve his country during the Great War (1914–18). A medical graduate from the University of Aberdeen in 1895, Gray was Consultant Surgeon to Aberdeen Royal Infirmary from 1904 till the outbreak of the war, when he volunteered for overseas service to put his surgical skills to military use. He spent more than three years in France, at first in charge of a group of base hospitals in Rouen and then as Consulting Surgeon to the British Third Army.

In the early months of the conflict, the management of war wounds was hopelessly inadequate. Filthy wounds caused by bullets or fragments of high explosive shell casing were contaminated by soil from the richly fertilised fields of France and Flanders containing the lethal organisms responsible for tetanus and gas gangrene. Casualties were often dealt with in field ambulances close to the front line, where their wounds were treated by superficial disinfection and suturing, before they were sent to base hospitals on or near the French coast for definitive surgical management. The journey sometimes took several days and patients reached base hospitals far too late, with established and overwhelming wound infections caused by pus forming organisms and by bacteria responsible for gas gangrene which often resulted in loss of limb or life. Gray was the first consulting surgeon during the war to describe wound excision, which is an operation to remove all devitalised tissue and foreign material in a systematic fashion till only healthy bleeding tissue remains.[1] This procedure was absolutely fundamental to the practice of war surgery and had to be performed as soon as possible after the infliction of a wound to reduce the risk of infection and to improve the chances of survival. Gray's work made a major contribution to urgent definitive surgery being performed in casualty clearing stations which were much closer to the front line than base hospitals and therefore reached more quickly. As a result, many lives were saved. Wound excision remains as important today as it was then.

Gray also developed expertise in the management of musculoskeletal wounds and was particularly noted for his treatment of compound fractures of the femur (thigh bone).[2] He documented an 80% mortality for this wound in 1914 and 1915.[3] In the early months of the war, these fractures were splinted inadequately and uncontrolled movement of the bones at the fracture site resulted in excessive blood loss. Most of the wounded reached casualty clearing stations in a state of circulatory collapse and were unlikely to survive. Gray ensured that all fractures of the femur were immobilised much more effectively, as a result of which wounded soldiers reached casualty clearing stations in a stable clinical condition and fit to undergo wound excision. The mortality rate was reduced to 15.6%. This was probably the most important surgical development to take place during the Great War.

---

1 Butler, A.G., *Official History of the Australian Army Medical Services, 1914–1918 Volume II – The Western Front*. Canberra: Australian War Memorial, 1940, p. 316.
2 A compound fracture is when the skin and muscles are breached right down to the fracture site. In war wounds, a penetrating bullet or shell fragment damages the skin and muscle before hitting the bone and shattering it. Clothing and debris from the battlefield carrying dangerous and sometimes lethal bacteria are driven into the depths of the wound.
3 Watson, F., *The Life of Sir Robert Jones*, London: Hodder & Stoughton, 1934, p. 158.

Although Gray was best known for his management of musculoskeletal wounds, his broad based knowledge and experience enabled him to deal with every type of wound. He even removed a bullet from the heart of a patient under local anaesthetic. He was acknowledged to be one of the most capable 'hands on' military surgeons of his era. Memoranda issued by Gray concerning the management of specific wounds were used by the British Third Army for which he was directly responsible from 1917, and were also available for the guidance of medical personnel in the other four British Armies in France and Flanders, who were given the opportunity to attend fracture courses organised and run by Gray.[4] Since he was such a leading authority, his courses were well attended. Towards the end of the war he wrote a book entitled *The Early Treatment of War Wounds*,[5] which epitomised the advancing knowledge of the period and which was aimed at inexperienced young medical officers going out to France and Flanders for the first time.

Gray returned to Aberdeen after being demobilised in 1919, but he never settled. In 1923 he was invited to take up the position of Surgeon-in-Chief to the Royal Victoria Hospital in Montreal, a prestigious position which usually carried high office with McGill University. He visited Montreal, where he met the Principal and Vice-chancellor, Sir Arthur Currie, who had led the Canadian Corps in France and Flanders most successfully during the final eighteen months of the war. History has judged Currie to be one of the most capable commanding officers to have served. Unfortunately, Currie had not been told about Gray's visit to Montreal and declared emphatically that Gray could not be guaranteed a University appointment. Despite this warning, Gray resigned from his position in Aberdeen and left for Montreal, where he became embroiled in

---

4 Carberry, A.D., *The New Zealand Medical Services in the Great War*. Auckland: Whitcombe and Tombs Ltd, 1924, p. 399.
5 Gray, H.M.W., *The Early Treatment of War Wounds*. London: Henry Frowde and Hodder & Stoughton, 1919.

bitter political infighting between Sir Arthur Currie and Sir Henry Vincent Meredith, President of the Royal Victoria Hospital. Rather than furthering his surgical prospects, the move to Montreal destroyed him professionally. There began a bizarre series of events which are still known to this day as the 'Sir Henry Gray Affair'[6] which culminated in his forced resignation and professional disgrace. He lived out the rest of his life in Montreal in surgical obscurity.

This biography provides the reader with a full account of the many factors in Gray's family background which helped to form and shape his personality. It deals with his surgical career, beginning with his early days in Aberdeen when he established himself as an outstanding surgeon. It goes on to describe his many achievements during the war years when his contributions were of enormous importance and ends with the most controversial phase of his life in Montreal. It then looks back over his career, analysing the strengths which made Gray such an outstanding surgeon and the weaknesses which contributed to his downfall. It is one hundred years since Henry Gray established the principles of modern war surgery, yet hardly anyone in his home city of Aberdeen knows of him. The authors hope that this account of his life will help to restore his name to somewhere near its rightful place.

---

6 Hanaway, J., R. Cruess, J. Darragh, *McGill Medicine Volume 2, 1885–1936*. Montreal: McGill-Queen's University Press, 2006, pp.112–113.

CHAPTER 2

Gray's Family Background

Henry McIlltree Williamson Gray was born on 14 March 1870, at 2 Rosemount Terrace, Aberdeen, the fifth child of Alexander Reith (A.R.) Gray and Barbara Shand Anderson.

The couple married on 20 August 1863, in Aberdeen, and lost their first child, Robert, to diphtheria at the age of three weeks in 1864. Henry was thus fourth in line after Alexander (Aleck) Reith (b.1866), William Anderson (b.1867) and Barbara Begg (b.1868). In 1872 his sister, Jane Reith (known as Jeannie) arrived, followed by Alice Robina in 1873 (d.1874) and Adam in 1875. Eight years later, his parents would have what effectively became a 'second family' when John was born in 1882, and Eva Esther in 1885.

Henry Gray was very much the son of both his parents. So many of the character traits that constituted his complex personality he shared with them. Their pleasant disposition, industriousness, diligence and perseverance were all discernible in him to varying degrees, whilst his father's impulsiveness and propensity for risk taking and his mother's unassuming manner and fortitude were also a part of his makeup. Moreover, the principles of honesty, loyalty and the value of hard work they upheld were instilled in him and his siblings from an early age. Indeed, from the considerable information that has been passed down either through letters or by word of mouth about A.R. Gray and Barbara Anderson and the kind of people they were, qualities as well as shortcomings can be glimpsed that would later contribute to making Henry Gray the person he was.

Henry's father took nothing for granted. Born in Old Meldrum, Aberdeenshire on 2 October 1830, to crofters, Adam and Jane Reith Gray, he was the eldest of five children, whom the 1841 Census lists as four sons Alexander, Robert, Adam, James, and a daughter, Elspet.

Whilst his parents eeked out a living on the land, the hardscrabble existence into which the children were born was made bearable by the roles played by both church and school in their lives. Henry's paternal grandparents were respectable people and staunch churchgoers who were able to read and write in a simple fashion, but could not afford to offer their children anything more than a very basic education. A.R. Gray must have realised quite early on that if he were ever to be more than a semi literate farm labourer, he would need to improve himself way beyond that point. And he was not alone. Robert, his younger brother by two years, would have faced the same challenges for he too rose above their farming background to become an army surgeon. It is not known how they managed, coming as they did from such humble beginnings, but it is certain that their upbringing was a very far cry from the privileged one Henry would enjoy thirty years later. Indeed, without much more than a family bible in the home, they would have had to use every available means by which to glean an education, namely, Sunday school, bible study, the village schoolroom and frequent independent study of the scriptures and classics. Perhaps, as gifted and hardworking schoolboys eager for knowledge, they came to the notice of a kindly minister or school mistress who lent them books and encouraged their studies. Whatever means these sons of poor crofters used to obtain an education, their achievement was remarkable.

A.R. Gray and his brother acquired a level of literacy and culture that would eventually secure them a place in society as 'gentlemen', something Henry and his brothers would later consider their birthright. Letters exchanged between his father and his uncle in 1860, when Robert was an army medical officer in India, are eloquent, their elegant, unfussy writing showing an innate grasp of language and propriety. Particularly commendable is the fact that these personal letters are written without recourse to any of the clichés and the flowery biblical language beloved by so many Victorians of the elder Grays' background. They mirror those between Henry and his siblings written many years later that display a natural

FIGURE 2.1
Alexander Reith Gray, c 1888

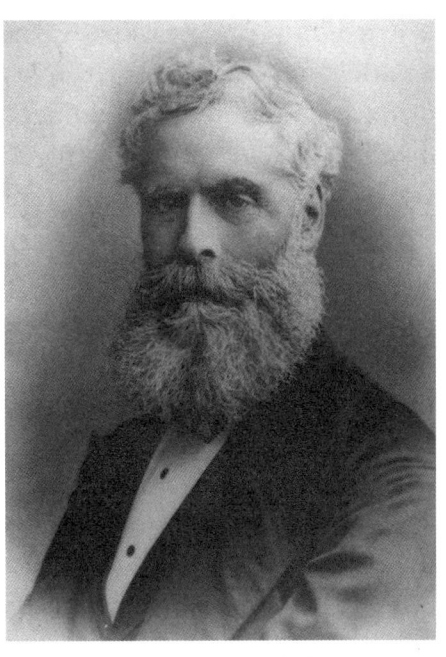

ease with writing and sophisticated word play. A.R. Gray's eventual ascent to the position of prominent Aberdeen citizen and highly successful business man, and Robert's career as a respected surgeon, came about through single-mindedness and a dogged determination to succeed that was not deterred by adversity. A.R. Gray would later attach great importance to the schooling of his own children, including his daughters, for they all without exception benefitted from the very best education available.

In spite of their success family records reflect that whilst Henry's father and uncle were ambitious men who were determined to improve themselves and better their lives, they never turned their backs on the people they left behind and their humble origins. They kept in touch with their parents in Old Meldrum, and mention is made of them in their letters. A.R. Gray gave jobs to his younger brothers while both he and Robert helped support their father when, after the death of his wife in 1860, he left his farm and came to live in Aberdeen with his niece, Margaret Gray Skene. These facts serve as evidence of the strength of the family ties that existed between the Grays at the time. Moreover, the sense of responsibility they felt towards relatives, was later instilled in the children of Henry's generation and passed down.

Henry's mother, Barbara Anderson, was eighteen when she

married thirty-two year old A.R. Gray. At the time she was living in a middle-income part of town at 7 Forbes Street with her mother, maternal grandmother and three of her siblings, her father having died in 1857. According to the 1861 Census two years earlier, the family owned the property. If not exactly a beautiful girl, Barbara was attractive, good humoured, quiet and agreeable. She was also young and healthy, important assets in a prospective wife at the time, particularly given the Victorian propensity for large families. The daughter of a master builder, William Anderson, who had grown prosperous enough to purchase (or perhaps build) his own house, Barbara had benefitted from a genteel upbringing and a good education for a middle class girl of the day. Like A.R. Gray, she came from a devout Presbyterian background, and importantly for him she was not so elevated socially that she would look down on his humbler origins.

Henry's parents met in 1862 at the Bon Accord Free Church, then located in the Gaelic Chapel on Gaelic Lane, and their courtship lasted for about a year. As was the custom of the day, it was conducted mainly through chaperoned meetings between them in her family's drawing room and by correspondence. From the forty-six letters Henry's father wrote to his mother during this period that have survived to this day and which she kept in a rosewood sewing box, it is evident that whilst he was an ardent and persistent suitor, she was not always so encouraging. Although none of her letters to him were kept after his death, she is reflected through his as being a gentle, reserved young woman who was wise beyond her years and not in any hurry to get married. Whatever the cause of her reticence, it is evident from the way he writes and comments on her behavior that she did not share his ability to express her feelings. It is impossible to read one of the letters without being struck by the dichotomy between the palpable spontaneity and openness of Henry's father and the relatively undemonstrative nature of his mother as reflected through him. Henry's father's letters are now over 150 years old, but they are a charming witness to the sincerity of his feelings, the uprightness of his character and the universal nature of his plight. Tenderness and humour run side-by-side anxiety and apprehension. For if in Barbara he felt he had found a soul mate, and he clearly did – albeit a much younger one – he was not always confident in his ability to persuade her to be his wife. It was a situation made all the more tantalizing by the fact that he felt himself to be so right for her. And there is no doubt that he was an eligible bachelor. Not only was he a committed churchman, which would have been essential for his acceptance into the Anderson family, his letters also reflect a man of good character who was personable, kind and highly driven. Furthermore, judging by his photograph presumably taken in his fifties, he was handsome- an asset perhaps not entirely lost on his intended. In 1857 he had set himself up as a general merchant employing his younger brother by eight years, James, as a clerk. By 1863 he is recorded on the couple's marriage certificate as a Commission Merchant, which would seem to indicate that he was acting as an agent or broker, although it is not clear in exactly which field of commodities. At all events, he now saw himself as established and able to take care of a wife and family.

Before his marriage, A.R. Gray had been living in a working class area at 39 Affleck Street where, according to the same census, he and James were lodgers, renting two rooms in a small terraced house from their cousin, Margaret, and brother-in-law, John Skene, a carter by trade. Altogether there were ten people in residence, four adults and six children, two of whom aged ten and thirteen were servants. There is little doubt that A.R. Gray would have been relieved to find an alternative solution to his living arrangements and the prospect of setting up home with Barbara would have been an attractive one. They started out life together in quite modest accommodation at 135 Crown Street, just around the corner from Affleck Street, and it was at the same address that three-week old Robert died a year later. Soon after this misfortune, when Barbara was expecting Aleck, the couple moved to Rosemount Terrace, a rather better neighborhood, where Henry was born five years later.

Barbara was twenty-four when she gave birth to Henry. At the time the Grays were living in decent though not lavish accommodation, with limited domestic help that included a cook and a nursemaid for the children. The competition would have been strong with four children under five vying for their mother's attention and Henry would not remain the baby of the family for very long. Like the three older children, he had to cede his position to several younger ones in quick succession. Henry was two years old when Jeannie was born and the family moved to more spacious surroundings at 15 North Silver Street.

Barbara Gray bore ten children in twenty-one years, which was not uncommon for the times, and eight of them were born in the first eleven years of her marriage. Perhaps less usual was that in an age when fathers tended to be somewhat distant from their offspring, particularly during infancy, delegating the care of them essentially to their wives and servants, A.R. Gray was said to have been exceptionally fond of his children to the point of being actively involved in their lives. In spite of a very demanding workload as his business expanded, he spent time with them and particularly enjoyed playing with the babies of his growing family. This is a trait that Henry would inherit from his father, for he too would show great interest and pride in his own children, reporting their development enthusiastically to his mother and siblings in conversations recorded later by his youngest sister, Eva, in her journals.

On 14 December 1874 the family suffered a blow when Alice, a hitherto healthy toddler, died of what is recorded on her death entry as 'croup lasting fourteen days'. Although the loss of a child was a very common occurrence in Victorian Britain and families were generally accepting of it, Eva, the youngest Gray, remembered from remarks her mother later made that the deaths of first Robert and then Alice were keenly and equally felt by both their parents. How much the Gray children were shielded at the time from their grief at losing one year old Alice has not been documented and their parents were nothing if not stoic and dutiful, but there is little doubt that her sudden absence would have been felt by them all. Henry was four when Alice died and Jeannie was barely two. Eleven months later when their mother gave birth to Adam, the focus of her attention would again be on another baby. During a period of time when the entire family was surrounded by loss and change, Henry would be particularly vulnerable due to his position in the family. Too old to be treated like a baby, yet not quite old enough to be able to rationalize his own feelings and those of others, he would have been struggling to make his needs known. Indeed, so many adjustments in such a short space of time would be considered an intolerable burden for any four-year-old today. The Grays, however, were evidently what would be regarded now as their own very efficient support group. From what is known of Henry's parents, it was clearly through their staunch religious belief, which pervaded every aspect of their lives that they managed to comfort each other, surmount their grief and give an example of courage to their children. Like many a devout Victorian family, their faith was their solace in the face of misfortune, and they drew on it freely. The Scriptures were read at meal times, passages were learned and frequently invoked – some were copied painstakingly onto sheets of paper that were later found tucked into family bibles and prayer books. The children were encouraged to examine their consciences in the light of what they had learned and pray daily. It was thus natural for them to resort to prayer in time of need.

Journals left by Eva, written at the age of twelve in 1897 and between the ages of twenty and twenty-two from 1905–7, are full of lighthearted girlish enthusiasm reflecting a happy, privileged lifestyle spent in the company of a loving family and close friends. In spite of the easygoing nature of each entry, however, frequent mention is made of churchgoing; sermons are discussed and preachers rated, while she occasionally takes herself to task for being uncharitable or too worldly in her outlook.

If Henry and his siblings, from eldest to the youngest, were taught to value honesty and loyalty, they also shared a strong sense of personal responsibility. Letters exchanged between them in adulthood speak to a rectitude and a caring for others that it would be hard to

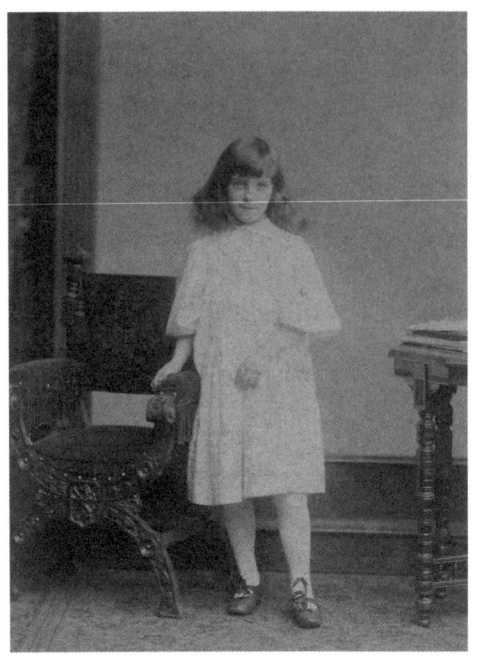

FIGURE 2.2
Eva Esther Gray in 1890 aged five.

better. It was this strict moral upbringing that would mark Henry for life and form the bedrock of his own life-work ethic.

In 1865 A.R. Gray would face what was probably the most challenging time of his professional life when he was forced to declare bankruptcy. Two years after his marriage to Barbara and a year after the death of their firstborn, Robert, when great joy had turned suddenly to tragedy, this single event more than any other would inform the last twenty-four years of his life – and in a subtle way those of his children. Henry was born five years later, but he and his siblings all grew up in the knowledge of what had befallen their father. Little is known of the circumstances under which the crisis occurred. It was reported in the *London Gazette* on 17 March 1865, and three men trusted him sufficiently to come forward to underwrite the debt. One of them, a Mr Williamson, may have been a close friend, since Henry appears to have been named after him. A.R. Gray subsequently signed a promissory note, undertaking to repay them over a period of twelve years. And he kept his word. On 1 August 1877, he wrote a letter to his creditors saying the time had come for him to make good the debt, and he surprised them all by including interest at two and a half percent on the sum borrowed, which, according to Eva, they had not expected. Through this unfortunate event A.R. Gray not only instilled in his children a respect for the dictum that 'a gentleman's word is his bond' and that monies lent must be repaid, he also taught them about the true cost of money and fairness in business, even between friends. Found amongst Eva's belongings after her death in 1968 was a pristine copy of that letter, which she had kept wrapped up in yellowing tissue paper as a memento of her father's scrupulous honesty and determination to overcome his financial difficulties. Although the crisis had occurred twenty years prior to her birth, she was proud of the memory of his achievement and would sometimes remind her children and grandchildren of it as an example of perseverance in the face of despondency and failure. The story of A.R. Gray's struggle and shame from which he emerged triumphant, thanks to his friends and his own hard work, was thus passed down through the generations. In fact, it is still sometimes referred to by his descendants, because it is as relevant today as it has ever been.

With A.R. Gray's bankruptcy had come the realisation that he must change direction. It was no good thinking he could continue to trade as a general merchant or a mere broker. If he wanted to succeed, it would take much more than that and he set about finding a solution. He needed to develop a new business model. He must come up with something that no one else had thought of doing before and he used all of his innate entrepreneurial skills and experience to find it. In his twenties, A.R. Gray had travelled widely in India, Pakistan and Afghanistan as a representative for medical suppliers to the British Army. He had also lived briefly in the Cape Colony as a would-be settler. It is likely that both experiences would have exposed him to a variety of exotic foodstuffs that did not exist in Aberdeen, because it was on these that he came to focus his enquiry. In fact, he simply did what any successful high-end entrepreneur has always done. First he identified what wealthy people could not obtain without his help and then he convinced them that they needed it. In the absence of refrigeration, he created a luxury food business specializing in such delicacies of the day as imported tinned peaches and pineapple; exotic chutneys and jams; specialty tea, coffee and fine wine. He also sold aged Scotch whisky and developed a market for it abroad. In order to bring all these luxuries under one roof, he opened a shop in his name in the centre of Aberdeen, although the firm's headquarters remained at Upper Market, Union Street. A.R. Gray then worked tirelessly to attain his goal and the profits from the new business went from strength to strength. They subsequently soared and by 1877 he had become very prosperous. Known affectionately as 'the man who brought tinned peaches to Aberdeen', he had literally become a legend in his own lifetime. Until the 1980s his name was still painted on the wharf of the harbour in Aberdeen, a sign of the volume of commercial activity he had generated for well over a century. And a company by the name of A.R. Gray still trades in foodstuffs to this day, although it no longer belongs to the family.

In 1877 when Henry was seven, his father commissioned a large house to be built at 9, Queen's Road, Aberdeen, where he would live for the rest of his life. From that point on he and his family enjoyed a privileged lifestyle and he was able to educate his children in a befitting manner. He began by having them expertly privately tutored and then one by one sent them to prestigious boarding schools. Merchiston Castle School in Edinburgh (established 1830) was selected for the boys and Roedeen School in Brighton (established 1885) for Jeannie and later, Eva. Their elder sister, Barbara (b.1868), was probably educated at home and in Aberdeen, since Roedeen would not have existed when she was of school age.

In 1884, when Henry Gray was fourteen, he was sent to join his elder brother, William, then seventeen, at Merchiston Castle School. He would remain there until 1888. Aleck, A.R. Gray's eldest son who was two years older than William, had left the school at the age of sixteen in 1881 to be groomed for his father's business, having shown signs of exceptional business acumen, but little interest in undertaking further studies. William, on the other hand, was a particularly outstanding student whose ambition it was to pursue a university education and study medicine. He set the bar high for Henry who was doubtless aware of the challenge that lay ahead as the younger brother of a very bright pupil. The school has no academic record of Henry, since the campus moved some miles from its original location in 1930 and the relevant archives are no longer available. Nevertheless, the school magazine, 'The Merchistonian', has survived for the period 1886–88 and reports that he was made a prefect in 1888, his final year at Merchiston. At the end of that year, Henry passed the routine examinations required for university entrance, which strongly implies that he was in good academic standing with the school.

The Merchistonian also makes some interesting observations regarding Henry's prowess as a sportsman. He excelled at both rugby and cricket. For the 1886–87 season he is reported in the rugby section as being a forward weighing in at 11 stone 5¼ pounds and it goes on to describe his performance in the following terms: 'indefatigable in the front, where he is always to be found. Has done splendid work, and shone in many a rush. Dribbles well, and is a strong tackler'. By all accounts he was a natural cricketer, as well as a particularly talented bowler. In the 'School Gossip' section of the same edition the writer notes:

> Of the bowlers, Gray stands in a class apart, and would find a place in any Public School eleven. He always bowls a good length with considerable spin from the off and, when things are going wrong, knows how to keep his head and his temper . . . His record up to the present of 62 wickets for under 6 runs a piece speaks for itself, and he should have little difficulty in surpassing his performance of last year.

Reporting on the 'Characters of the Eleven' in 1888, when Henry was captain of the cricket team, there is an insightful analysis of him that would seem to transcend mere cricket in its description of his temperament and his interaction with the rest of the team. Henry is said to possess a 'suavity of manner and the imperturbability of temper that help things to run smoothly and prevent friction'. These were early signs of an ability to communicate effectively and calmly under stressful conditions – to keep his head during anxious moments, and to win the admiration of others for the elegant way in which he acquitted himself. In fact, 'suavity of manner and imperturbability of temper' were hallmarks of the Gray family. All the children of Henry's generation inherited their parents' amiability and poise. Moreover, the good-natured personal qualities that sprang from this legacy made them very likeable people.

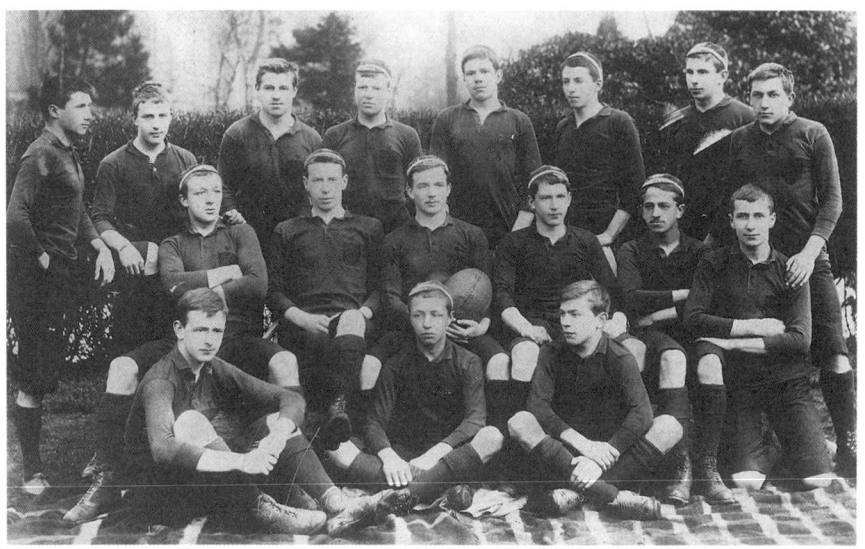

FIGURE 2.3
Merchiston Castle 1st XV, 1888, Merchiston Castle School, Edinburgh. Henry Gray is centre front.

When Henry left Merchiston in 1888, he did not go straight to university. Instead, he went to work for his father. The family business was still continuing to grow and prosper and A.R. Gray would have been proud to have another of his sons join the firm. It is not known exactly what prompted Henry to do so, but he spent the next two and a half years there, picking up the rudiments of business practice along the way. His subsequent decision to change course and pursue a university education came in 1891, and it happened to follow his brother William's death from 'croupous pneumonia' at the age of twenty-four, a condition that, according to his death entry, lasted five days. In all probability, this would have been pneumococcal pneumonia, a very serious condition in the pre-antibiotic era. William was a second year medical student at Edinburgh University, having previously graduated with an MA in Classics from Balliol College, Oxford. He died on 11 April at home in Aberdeen during the Easter vacation. Eva Gray was six when this occurred, but in spite of her young age she could remember her brother well and always spoke of him with great affection. Eva's daughter, Helen Leach, remembers her mother describe William as a 'saintly' character who was beloved by all who knew him. Eva also spoke of the profound sadness his death had caused her parents and indeed, the entire family. Significant, perhaps, is the fact that although A.R. Gray had hitherto registered the births and deaths of his children himself, it is Henry's signature that appears on William's death entry.

Whether Henry's decision to train as a doctor was prompted directly by William's death is not known. The idea that it was is a compelling one, coming as it does at such a key moment in his professional development. William had been such an exemplary person and so outstanding a student – and his loss so painful – that Henry with typical filial loyalty may very well have felt the urge to take his place. Henry, however, is recorded as telling his friend, John Christie, in September 1891, that 'he was not suited for a career in business' and that he was going to register for medical school that autumn, so he may also have been contemplating a change before his brother died. The likelihood is that Henry had been bored for a while with what he was doing and that William's death made him re-examine his life in the light of something new. Motivated as he may have been to do justice to William's memory, the outstanding excellence he achieved first as a medical student and later as a surgeon, remains a tribute to Henry alone.

After William's death, A.R. Gray became progressively incapacitated by exhaustion and ill health. Eva would later describe her father as 'a kind and good man' who had 'worked himself to death', but she conceded that it was unlikely that overwork alone could be held responsible for his condition. By the end of 1891 it was becoming increasingly difficult for him to keep normal office hours and he was depending heavily on Aleck to take over the day-to-day running of the business.

A brief moment of happiness brightened the early part of 1892 for the Grays when Barbara, aged twenty-four, married John Stewart on 4 February and Jeannie, aged twenty, married Howard Coote, on 24 April. Both girls might be said to have married 'well', having chosen charming men of impeccable character with enough money to see them live comfortably – and Jeannie rather more so than Barbara. For while John was established in his career as the Manager of the Bank of Scotland in Aberdeen and could provide amply for a wife and family, Howard came from a distinguished family of landowners in Huntingdonshire and had inherited considerable wealth.

After his elder daughters left home, A.R. Gray's condition continued to deteriorate. Then, when the family was least expecting it, Barbara died on 22 February 1893. One month earlier on 17 January, she had given birth to a daughter, Barbara Constance. This sad event was very clearly remembered by Eva who, at eight, was old enough to feel the full impact of Barbara's death. Suddenly all the excitement over her sister's marriage and the arrival of the new baby had been overturned. She was seventeen years younger than Barbara, but they had been close. Years later she would remember her with tears in her eyes as 'a sweet thing' and 'a most loving person'. Little Barbara Constance, who was brought up by her father and his family, spent holidays with the Grays and Eva kept in touch with her off and on all her life.

The shock and grief of losing Barbara was made all the more agonising by the fact that A.R. Gray's condition suddenly took a marked turn for the worse. He began to exhibit completely uncharacteristic bouts of moodiness and angry outbursts that greatly alarmed his wife and older children, and terrified the younger ones. His pleasant demeanor became clouded with furious religious ranting alternating with expressions of the utmost sadness and despair, all of which left him feeling ever more debilitated. Although there is no surviving correspondence between the siblings referring to A.R. Gray's illness, Eva remembered that this was a very sad period for the entire family. The situation was made all the more difficult by the fact that no one really knew what was wrong with him. Henry, who by 1894 was in his last year of medicine, was in all probability living away from home, but he would have seen his father whenever he came to visit and he would have witnessed the deterioration in his health. It is not known how much Henry was involved in trying to find a cure for his father, but it is likely that he had some contact with the family doctor who advocated an extended stay abroad. Eventually a decision was made to take A.R. Gray to Rotorua in New Zealand, well known for its spa, where it was hoped the waters would be beneficial to his health. In March 1894 he sailed for Wellington with his wife and the two youngest children, John and Eva. They also took along with them a tutor who is named on the passenger list as 'Mr G.A. Anderson', and may possibly have been a relative of Barbara Shand Gray (nee Anderson).

On 31 August 1894, A.R. Gray died aged sixty-three, one month before his sixty fourth birthday. He had suffered from progressive impairment of cerebral function for three years. Perhaps he had severe cerebro-vascular disease, leading to multiple brain infarcts. He may have had early onset dementia, or a brain tumour, but his symptoms had been present for three years, which is a long time for a tumour. A primary malignant brain tumour would have certainly caused his death much more quickly, so any growth would have to have been at the benign end of the spectrum. In accordance with his dying wish, the family made the long journey back to Scotland with his remains. They were met en route in London by Henry and his uncle Robert, the two doctors of the family, who signed the appropriate papers and accompanied the family back to Aberdeen. A.R. Gray was interred in the 'family burying ground' at Nellfield Cemetery beside Robert, Alice and William, where Barbara Shand Gray was buried in 1908 and Aleck in 1946. Barbara Begg Gray Stewart's grave is close by.

While anything that is known about Henry's personal life comes chiefly through his letters to Eva and the memories she subsequently shared with her family, her four journals were also a significant source of information about him. That of 1897, written at the age of twelve in pencil on a large commercial calendar advertising life insurance, is charming and funny. It recounts enthusiastically her day to day life at 9 Queen's Road just before she, John and their mother moved to a smaller house – *The Gables* in Rubislaw Den South – in another comfortable area of Aberdeen. Eva, who is clearly not a spoilt child, is nonetheless much cherished and her view of the world reflects this richly. Her sense of fun is apparent and delightful. There is the feeling that memories of sad events have long since been swept away and there is a refreshing lightness in the way she records the passing of time. In amongst the daily entries about family, friends, school, music lessons, homework, church and meals that have a tendency to repeat themselves with exasperating regularity, there are amusing anecdotes. This was the year that Henry married Katherine Anne Rattray, known to all as 'Kate', on 27 October, and their names come up often, chiefly with reference to picnics and outings, though not exclusively so. One entry on 30 July depicts Henry in disgrace. It records how he lost the family dog he was supposed to be looking after for the day. It is probable that Henry was no longer living at home and that he had come round especially to feed it and take it for a walk while the others were out. At all events, he appears to have had his mind on other things, because he let it run off and the reader is left in no doubt as to Eva's views on the matter. For, as she remarks with affectionate exasperation in the face of Henry's inattention, it was only thanks to John's superior ability to find and catch the errant 'Villain' that he was ever seen again.

Eva was very fond of all her brothers, but it was with Henry, Adam and John that she had the most contact as a young girl and with whom she felt the closest bond at that time. Little is known of Adam after he emigrated to New Zealand at the age of eighteen in 1893 to work with a sheep farmer who was a distant relative. Eva felt his

Gray's Family Background

absence keenly at the time and kept in contact with him sporadically over the years. The family did meet up with him again in 1894 while they were there seeking a cure for his father and according to Eva he eventually made a good life for himself, but he never seems to have returned to Scotland and there is no mention of him in any of Henry's letters to her. Aleck, who was now married to Janet with two children, had taken on the role of father figure. He was now also head of the family business, and watched over his siblings' incomes and investments; Eva thus looked to him more as provider than brother. Aleck was, however, very affectionate towards his younger sister, as was Janet, and many letters survive from them that attest to their care and concern for her.

The months of January and February are missing, doubtless due to wear and tear given the age of the calendar, and some of the days have been skipped, but the diary remains a cohesive account of a happy late Victorian childhood spent in and around Aberdeen.

The journals then move to 1905/6 and 7, by which time Eva has grown into a young lady. In 1905 she was twenty and very popular with the young men in her entourage, although she often appears to find their attentions tiresome. Most of these were known to her through John via Merchiston and Sandhurst, but she also not surprisingly seems to have caused quite a stir amongst the young officers in India when she and her mother made the trip there to see John, then serving with the 36th Sikhs in Peshawar.

These were busy years for Henry who was building his career and his reputation in Aberdeen, but there are frequent references to him throughout these journals that indicate he was very much in touch with his sister at that time. Eva also met many people through her elder sister, Jeannie, now living in some style in

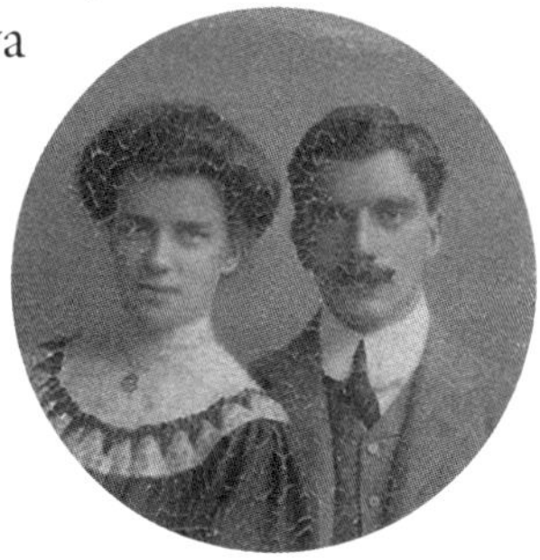

FIGURE 2.4
Eva and John Gray: c 1905.

Huntingdonshire. Jeannie's husband, Howard Coote, would eventually become Lord Lieutenant of the county. Howard was, by all accounts, a very likeable person with whom Henry and his siblings were always most friendly. Eva's life, which had always been materially very comfortable if a little limited socially, took an upward turn when she began to visit Jeannie and Howard regularly with her mother at Stukeley Hall. The Cootes were generous hosts and their hospitality was legendary. There was a constant flow of guests, with house parties, dinner parties, balls, hunting and bridge to keep everyone busy. Henry occasionally visited if he ever had to go down to London on business and he lent Howard his car when the Cootes came up on holiday to Scotland, so they could go touring.

Several letters from Henry to Eva have survived from this period and one in particular dated 27 May 1907, concerns amongst other things her brief hospitalization in Marseilles on her way back from India. The letter was sent to Stukeley where she was convalescing. No details of her condition are given, but Henry's tone is avuncular and comforting. 'I had a very good letter from the doctor at Marseilles giving me all the particulars which I wanted to hear', he writes. 'He seems to be a good and decent chap and probably quite correct about his opinions. I hope he will feel better after being thus patted on the back!' Henry's tone is mildly patronising and it is unclear why the said doctor needed to 'feel better' in the first place. Perhaps he was French but spoke very good English. If so, it was just as well since Henry's French was poor to say the least, although he did speak and write reasonable German.

After the death of her mother in 1908, Eva went to live permanently with her sister at Stukeley, returning to Aberdeen occasionally to stay with Henry and Aleck. Henry and Kate were particularly insistent that Eva join them as often as possible. 'Looking forward muchly to seeing you – but you have to stay practically all the time with us', Henry wrote enthusiastically on 25 October 1908, for she was extremely popular with their children and very good company for them all. In 1909 she made another trip to India to visit

John, where she became engaged to a young doctor, Ernest Simson, from Edinburgh nicknamed 'Kemo', a contemporary of her brother and an old Merchistonian. The couple were to be married the following year when he would be on leave in Scotland. The Grays were delighted with the match and thrilled to think of Eva finally settled at the age of twenty-five. Kemo was John's greatest friend and a charming man who clearly loved and respected their sister. He was also a good doctor who had earned Henry's approval, and a fine sportsman having played rugby for Scotland. Eva's joy was to be short-lived, however, for not long after her return to Britain news arrived that he had died of cholera. This was a devastating blow to a young woman who, in addition to experiencing such sorrow, had only recently lost her mother and her home in Aberdeen. The family immediately responded to the crisis with help and support. Jeannie and Howard were with her at Stukeley to comfort her, while Henry, John and Aleck were in close and frequent contact.

Henry and Kate had three children over six years starting with Katharine Eva, born in 1903. Esther Frances followed in 1905 and Henry Robert in 1906. They were by all accounts attentive and loving parents, who put their children first and were proud of their achievements, and they certainly earned the love and devotion of their offspring. Eva's 1905 journal mentions several visits to The Gables from two-year-old Katharine over that summer. This was six months or so after Esther was born when Kate would have been busy with the baby and relieved to have her toddler occupied. For although she had a good deal more help in the home than most people today, she and Henry were still very involved with their children, and their upbringing was not left to a nanny. Sometimes Henry comes for Katharine if he can get away early, as on 29 June when Eva also notes, 'Henry got his new car this afternoon and it is a ripper – all green – 18 h.p. – goes like a drink!!' This was probably the same car that the Aberdeen University magazine mentions in a tribute to Henry as a distinguished alumnus in 1905, where it declares rather solemnly, 'Mr Gray is an enthusiastic motorist, and is possessed of a thorough knowledge of the car he drives'. And while he certainly did take his motoring seriously, he also greatly enjoyed ferrying his children around and witnessing their excitement.

The following year on 14 May 1906, after Henry and Kate had moved to a larger property at Kingswells, Eva writes in evident delight:

> Katharine came in from Kingswells to spend the day – arrived with Henry in car at 9 am and left at 5. Perfectly sweet and contented all day dear wee kiddy. Took her to see Aunties A and J. She is a darling and so entertaining.

In a letter to Eva dated 27 December 1906, when she was in India with her mother visiting John, Henry delivers an endearingly detailed and funny account of the family's Christmas morning experience that has universal resonance; fortunately for the family, Kate's sister, Molly, was staying.

> Christmas passed amidst great excitement on the part of the family. Esther woke up at 2.30 am! Molly kept her going till 6.30 when she carried her to our room and she was propped up between Kate and me. Then remarks, increasing in loudness gradually, were made about stockings and Kang suddenly showed signs of life and was bolt upright and wide awake. Then there was no more sleep that morning! The whole family have been simply overloaded with gifts of all sorts. The nursery looks like a toyshop.

Esther's life was said to have taken a tragic turn when, at the age of about nine months she managed to crawl into a doll's cot and then fall from it. She was subsequently noted to have a curvature of her spine and family history attributed the deformity to the fall. It is very likely, however, that this incident drew attention to a pre-existing underlying abnormality. What is clear is that the deformity progressively increased throughout Esther's childhood causing difficulty with walking.

In that same Christmas letter Esther was exactly eleven months

FIGURE 2.5
Henry Gray taking delivery of a new car with Katharine and Esther at the back in bonnets, circa 1907

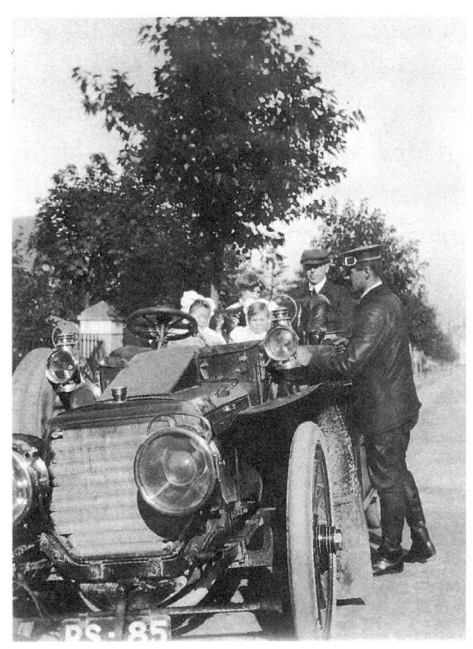

old and Henry goes on to comment, 'she has improved very much since we fixed her up and is as bright as possible except when possessed with outbursts of temper when her will is crossed in any way'. Of three-year-old Katharine (Kang) and Henry Junior who at four months old at the time was probably not sleeping through the night, he writes with characteristic humour, 'The boy is improving although Kate does not think so. Kang is in robust health and spirits – comes round with me in the car'.

Henry and Kate were not only loving parents, they also enjoyed spending time with their children, watching them play and develop. Old photographs from Barbara Shand Gray's album, many of which are sadly too faded now for publication, show uninhibited scenes of family picnics at the beach and amongst the heather – gatherings where the laughter and enjoyment are palpable. Henry and Kate are there watching over their children, refreshingly unperturbed by what might be happening to Katharine and Esther's long white dresses and Henry Junior's sailor suit. In another series of pictures from circa 1907/8, all three children play rowdily in the garden, rolling around on the lawn at *The Gables* – or perhaps it is Kingswells – the tea things scattered untidily on the grass as Henry and Kate look on indulgently. These photographs, likely taken by Eva and John who were keen photographers, are as full of atmosphere as they are amateurish. Not only do they bear witness to a rather more easy-going side to Edwardian childhood than one is used to reading about, they also hint at the kind of parents Henry and Kate were, in an age when children were still expected to be 'seen and not heard'. Here there is the sense that children must be allowed to be children and given the freedom to enjoy themselves. They should be loved and schooled, but not unduly fussed over. Later Henry and Kate's approach to parenting would be implicit in his letters to Eva whenever he wrote of his children's development – his humour and wisdom providing great comfort to her while bringing up a young family far away in India.

On 23 August 1913, twenty-seven year old Eva Esther Gray married thirty-two year old Harold Thomas Carew Ivens, (whom she calls Ivanhoe) a young captain in the 26th Punjabis. Their quiet wedding took place at St George's, Hanover Square. Eva had met Harold in India in 1909 and her fiancé 'Kemo' had been his friend. Harold wrote a letter of condolence to Eva upon Kemo's death, although he refrained from contacting her again for over a year. Their courtship took place while he was on leave in London. Their fifty-year marriage and the six children they had together were a source of great happiness and joy to them both. On 2 June 1914, Eva gave birth to her first child, Barbara Gray Ivens, in Hong Kong, where her husband was temporarily stationed.

Nine letters have survived from Henry to Eva for the period 1915–18, while he was in France and she in India. Full of family news, they also touch on deeper issues than in the past such as the ethical justification for the war and God's purpose for Europe, the ensuing mass destruction on the Western Front as well as in Mesopotamia, and the plight of the wounded, some of whom were known to them both from Aberdeen. This more sombre stance is partly due to the fact that the war has cast a pall over both their lives and they are moved to think more serious thoughts. However, whilst the war years engender a heightened sense of responsibility, they also seem to mark a coming of age for Eva in Henry's eyes. From this point on he considers her in a different light. It is as though she had responded to the call to be more thoughtful and surprised him. Increasingly there is the sense that he appreciates Eva's intelligence and her enquiring mind. He has realised that her interests are wide and certainly cannot be reduced to the mere bringing up of children, worthy though that may be. He still writes with the same easy affection, but she is now a match for him, an intellectual equal – and he never talks down to her unless it is to compensate with a self-deprecating quip he knows she will enjoy. Indeed, Eva had received a very good education for a young woman of her background at the turn of the 20th Century and she was also well read and informed all her life. For a short time before moving to England she had nursed beside her brother in Aberdeen and she had studied nursing in London for over a year with the intention of obtaining a qualification. Although she never regretted having chosen marriage and a family, her daughter, Helen Leach, remembers her mother saying that she would in some ways have liked an opportunity to stretch her intellectual abilities further. And with this subtle change in the way he perceives Eva, Henry realises that his detailed descriptions of the multiple operations he performs daily on wounded men will not be lost on her. There is thus no need to edit his words, to spare her the unpleasant details of battlefield casualties – of inflammation and pus, of shattered limbs and men dying from their appalling wounds in the mud and filth that was their living hell.

It is, however, when he writes about family and children to Eva that Henry's great capacity for tenderness and humour is most felt. This is in sharp contrast to the rather gruff exterior he often showed in the work place, particularly when challenged by someone he did not much care for.

1915 was the year Eva brought one-year old Barbara back to Aberdeen to meet the family for the first time and Henry, who has clearly been home on leave and seen her, is also delighted to relay the enthusiastic reports he has received from them all since his return. On 19 June he writes, 'Kate evidently thinks a tremendous lot of your little daughter Bretta – like I do'. Then with a word of warning, 'If she grows up to be like her mother she will do. So glad she is flourishing so well. Her mother will have to take care of her little self and not go lugging about her daughter too much'. On 10 August he notes of her visit to Aleck and Janet, 'You and Bretta seem to have made a great impression at Garthdee. Aleck writes very enthusiastically'.

A rather fatherly comment about Eva's wellbeing follows on 5 November when she is getting ready to return to India.

> Many thanks for your letter and for sending me the photo of yourself and your charming daughter. My word, she is looking well. Nearly as big as her mother. I hope she grows to be as good. I wish her mother were looking a bittie better than she is – an awful skinny malink still! You will have to take care of yourself my dear and don't go carrying about the daughter much.

On her journey back to India Eva thought she would be passing through Paris on her way to Marseilles to catch the boat. Unfortunately, Henry only found out at the last minute that he was able to get leave to travel to Paris to say goodbye, and their letters crossed. In fact, her train never stopped in Paris at all. Disappointed at missing her he writes:

> I am so sorry to have missed you after all. I got leave specially to come and see you . . . I hope you have a good journey. You will find a great stir at Marseilles from the embarkation of troops for Serbia . . . I thought I might see you at one of the Gares but Cook's people tell us that your special P & O does not actually come into Paris stations! Sickening.

On 27 February 1915, three months after Eva's return to India and shortly after little Barbara had had a bad bout of colic, Henry writes, 'So glad to hear that the wee daughter is well again. It was rotten for you and Ivanhoe. I hope you are both fit'.

On 13 March 1917, the day before his forty-seventh birthday, Henry sent a long letter from France to Eva in India full of news and comments about his family, although as ever the war continues to overshadow their lives. Esther was twelve at the time, while Katharine (nicknamed 'Kang') and Henry Junior were fourteen and eleven respectively. Of Esther he writes with evident concern:

> You will have heard, I have no doubt, that Esther has been having a poor time of it and had to be sent to the N. N. Home,[1] however last accounts are that she is ever so much better so I hope she will give no more anxiety poor kiddie. She has had a bad time of it all these years and deserves a good time in years to come – but God knows how this damned war will affect everyone and all one's own particular prospects and life.

Then with regard to the other two he notes rather more cheerfully,

> I get great letters from Katharine. She is developing into quite a modern young lady evidently. The boy also is at a very interesting stage and is going to turn out well I think. Kang and he have had mumps much to their annoyance, especially Kang's! who has been kept out of many important matters e.g. hockey matches and various exams!! She is also a very ardent Girl Guide.

Of Kate who was working hard for the war effort back in Aberdeen with a team of nurses, he reports not without a hint of exasperation, '(she) seems to be, as usual, doing too much. War dressings and teaching orderlies at Castlehill Barracks Hospital[2] and so on and so on. No use saying anything. Except for a usual winter bad cold however she seems to have kept in very good health.

In the same letter Henry is anxious to respond to news of Eva's two young children. He tells her how pleased he is to hear that one-

---

1 Possibly Nuffield Nursing Home.
2 From 1796, Gordon Highlanders were billeted in the Castlehill Barracks near the bottom of Union Street in Aberdeen. The Duke of Gordon founded the barracks on Castle Hill in 1794 with accommodation for 600 soldiers. In 1935, the Gordons left Castlehill for Bridge of Don Barracks.

year-old John is thriving, and asks after three-year-old Barbara. He wants to know whether she is still prone to the bouts of colic she has had in the past.

> Glad to hear such good reports of the family – that the boy is such a good chap – worthy of his parents. You say nothing of the wee daughter, or is she a thumping big girl now, having got over her tummy troubles again? I suppose she chatters all day long. Let's hear all about you all when you write, which please do soon.

But the war is ever present, and Henry is also concerned for Eva's husband, 'Ivanhoe', fighting in Mesopotamia. Particularly poignant for Henry and Eva was the fact that they had just lost their brother, John, in Mesopotamia the previous year. The circumstances of his tragic death and the impact it had on family members are discussed fully in Chapter 4.

On 13 March 1918, the day before his forty-eight birthday, Henry wrote to Eva in pencil from a congress of allied surgeons in France. He is sitting listening to speakers reading communications full of details that are 'laborious and tiring', so writing to her comes as a welcome distraction. This is Henry at his most light hearted as he chats away and jokes about some news she had sent him about her children, one aspect of which involves him. 'Delighted to hear such good accounts of your little ones', he says, 'but why you should laugh at wee "Jock" being so like his beautiful uncle I don't know – you should rather sympathize with him. The poor boy can't help the disability!' There is no doubt that he like everyone else is war weary, but he is ebullient as he contemplates the end of it, 'We are very quiet just now. Waiting for the great Boche attack which never comes[3] . . . He will get it in the neck if he does so in France'.

---

3 The Germans launched a massive offensive against the British 3rd and 5th Armies on 21 March 1918. 'Operation Michael' was an attempt to end the war before the United States could get sufficient numbers of men to France to bring about an allied victory, thanks to their unlimited resources.

After the war, in another letter to Eva in India, dated 14 April 1919, written just before the birth of her third child, Jane Isobel (the co-author's mother) on 17 April 1919 at the hill station of Naini Tal, Henry apologises for not having written for a while, and discusses his plans for the future after his upcoming demobilisation on 1 May. Given that he was so attentive towards Eva, it is ironic that he appears to have completely forgotten she was just about to give birth. This omission would have made her laugh heartily, however, and she would have forgiven him since at the time of writing he was convalescing from an operation (possibly to correct the neuritis in his left arm that had plagued him since his years in France). 'I was afraid that my neuritis was to play the deuce with me', he had written in 1917, 'but it causes practically no trouble now. I can just feel that all is not quite right in my left arm. It was beastly for nearly two years'. It seems likely that the trouble had returned and he could no longer live with the discomfort. Somewhat remarkable is that he was able to maintain the level of work demanded of him back in 1915 whilst in pain.[4]

Turning to fourteen-year-old Esther and her continuing difficulties, he writes:

> Esther is ever so much better. I think the mischief in her back is overcome but the unfortunate presence of a dislocated right hip mars her walking powers very seriously and pitiably. I hope something can be done to help her soon.

In addition to her spinal problem, Esther had developed a dislocated hip which made her disability very much worse and which greatly impaired her ability to walk. She had a pronounced limp which was painful. In later life, Esther was remembered by family members as having a very noticeable deformity of her spine and being extremely

---

4 He probably had a compression of one of the nerves (ulnar or median) supplying his hand which resulted in sensory loss in some of his fingers and also caused severe pain, which may have kept him awake at night.

restricted in her mobility. Perhaps the most likely explanation for Esther's spinal deformity and dislocated hip is a progressive neurological disorder resulting in very severe muscle imbalance. Such a provisional diagnosis is based solely on information provided by fragments of two letters from more than one hundred years ago and without further information about Esther's symptoms and physical signs, it is impossible to make a more precise diagnosis. Given these facts it is better to remain within the broad category of progressive neurological disorder and refrain from further speculation.

'The other two are flourishing', he writes of Katharine (sixteen) and Henry (thirteen). Then, clearly wanting to include Esther in some good news, he adds, 'all have developed extraordinarily in mental activity and you will be most amused and interested to see them again. I hope 1920 as you hint is possible'.

And of Kate whom his sister would also have wanted to hear about, he writes tenderly, '(she) is rather tired out after her strenuous war work of the past year. I hope she will pick up at Aboyne where they have meantime gone for a short time'.

Eva would indeed have been thrilled to have this news. She was a most nurturing person, and in spite of the distance between them and her preoccupation with the new baby, she would have revelled in hearing about Henry's family.

Five years later in 1922 when Eva loses her fourth child, Anne, aged sixteen months to diphtheria in India, Henry's response to his sister's tragic news (likely delivered by telegram) is tender and immediate.

> My dear 'lil' Eva', You know what a heap of sympathy is in the hearts of the household, one and all, with you and Harold and the kiddies. I got a great shock when I was told the news . . . God bless and comfort you all. It seems to me that we must feel little Anne's death only next to yourselves – and what is the good of saying anything more. God help you to bear your sorrow bravely as I am sure you try to do. I hope the others are all right and that you and Harold may be able to get away for a little all by yourselves, until the first great pangs of grief are over.

Suddenly, sick at heart and at a loss for more words, he ends the letter abruptly declaring, 'I don't feel inclined to write anything more. Your loving brother, Henry'.

Other letters written to Eva in 1927 and 1932, after the years of turmoil at McGill, reflect the same sense of comfort and security he has always felt in her presence. There is something of the old Henry in him again after a long period of disbelief and cynicism. There is talk of holidays and golf, of what their respective families are doing and the quality of his life in Canada. In the letter of 1932 he thanks Eva for 'the very interesting book' she has sent him for Christmas on German politics. He has not had time yet to read it properly, but he promises to do so soon. In spite of the rejection and disappointment he had suffered in Canada, there is the sense that they can still count on each other's loyalty.

It would be difficult to read Henry's letters to Eva without being struck by the very strong attachment that existed between them. They mirror her transition from adoring younger sister into something closely approaching 'confidante', as gradually she joins him in the role of devoted listener and valued sounding board. Their affection and admiration for each other, built on a mutual trust forged long ago out of sharing and loss, remained steadfast to the end. And it was surely this that prompted Kate to say in her letter comforting a grieving fifty-three year old Eva after his death in 1938, 'I know what your love for Henry IS'.

CHAPTER 3

Gray's career before the Great War

Gray's early career in Medicine

After completing his studies at Merchiston Castle School in Edinburgh in 1899, Henry Gray began working in his father's wholesale provision merchant's business. After two years, he decided he needed a change and as previously discussed, the death of his older brother William, in the spring of 1891 at the age of twenty four, may have been partly responsible for Gray's decision to study medicine. The reader will remember that William had been a second year medical student at the University of Edinburgh and had died of pneumonia. Gray also had a tendency to act on impulse and there is an account of him walking up Broad Street in Aberdeen where he met his friend John Christie heading purposefully in the direction of Marischal College, part of the University. Both men played cricket for Aberdeenshire. Christie had just completed his MA degree and when Gray asked Christie where he was going he learned that his friend was planning to enrol as a medical student. Gray announced that he would join him, saying that he was not cut out for a business career. So in October 1891 began the medical training of a man who was destined to become one of the most distinguished of Aberdonian surgeons.[1]

Gray graduated with honours in 1895. One of his medical classmates, in what was a very bright year, was Arthur Lister,[2] the nephew of Lord Lister, who had first introduced antiseptic surgery in 1865.

---

1 Porter, R.M.M., Recent Aberdeen Medical Teachers: Sir Henry Gray, KBE, CB, CMG, LLD, FRCS (Ed), *Aberdeen Postgraduate Medical Bulletin*, Oct. 1971, pp. 11–13.
2 Obituary, Sir Henry Gray. KBE, CB, CMG, LLD, FRCS (Ed), *British Medical Journal*, 15 October 1938, p. 814.

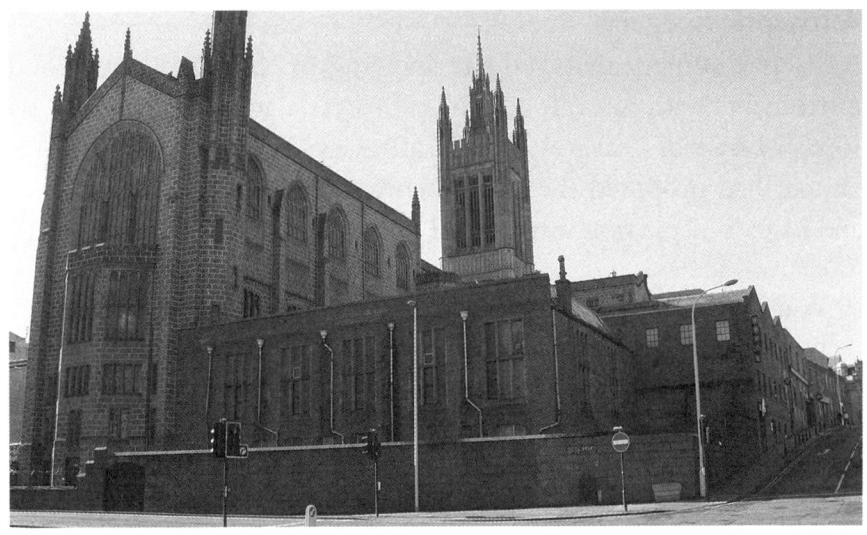

FIGURE 3.1
Marischal College, part of University of Aberdeen.

Gray's first appointment was house surgeon to Professor Sir Alexander Ogston, who is credited with bringing antiseptic surgery to Aberdeen, although perhaps he is best known for his 'discovery' of the staphylococcus, which was and still is, the most important micro-organism responsible for causing surgical wound infections.

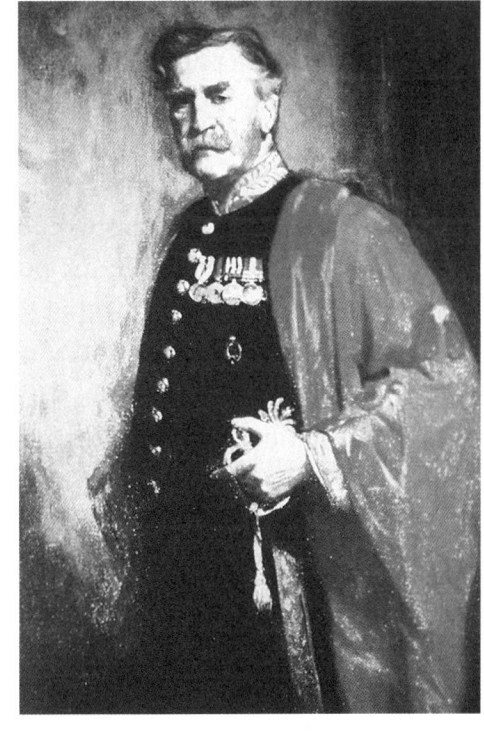

FIGURE 3.2
Portrait of Sir Alexander Ogston.

Antiseptic Surgery

Antiseptic surgery involved the spraying of surgical wounds and instruments with carbolic acid to kill bacteria and was first used by Joseph Lister at Glasgow Royal Infirmary in August 1865. Louis Pasteur had proposed the germ theory of disease the previous year and Lister's inspiration was derived from Pasteur's work. He declared:

> When it had been shown by the researches of Pasteur that the septic property of the atmosphere depended not on the oxygen or any gaseous constituent, but on minute organisms suspended in it, which owed their energy to their vitality, it occurred to me that decomposition in the injured part might be avoided without excluding the air, by applying as a dressing some material capable of destroying the life of the floating particles.[3]

The first patient to receive Lister's innovative treatment was a twelve year old boy admitted to Glasgow Royal Infirmary with a compound fracture of his tibia and fibula.[4] His leg had been run over by the wheel of a cart. Lister applied a pad of lint which had been soaked in carbolic acid to the boy's leg. After four days, he renewed the pad and discovered to his great delight that the wound looked clean and healthy. Without the dressing, the fracture would almost certainly have become infected and this would have resulted in delayed union of the broken bones. Happily, the boy's injury went on to rapid and uneventful healing with the help of the antiseptic dressing applied to the wound.[5] This case revolutionised surgical practice and soon

---

3 Lister, J., 'On the antiseptic principle in the practice of surgery.' *British Medical Journal*, 1867; 2: pp. 246–248.
4 The tibia and the fibula are the two bones in the leg between the knee and ankle. The term compound means that the broken bones in his leg had pierced the skin and had become contaminated with road dirt carrying bacteria to the fracture site. This is a particular problem with fracture of the tibia because it lies immediately beneath the skin with no intervening muscle and consequently readily becomes compound.
5 Lister, J., *op. cit.*

antiseptic surgery was being used widely. Lister went on to develop an elaborate dressing which consisted of a complex eight fold thick bandage of gauze treated with carbolic acid. There was a strip of mackintosh at the outer end of the dressing to act as a waterproof layer and an impermeable silk against the skin to protect the skin from the corrosive effects of the carbolic acid.[6]

Ogston was using antiseptic methods for his surgery when Gray was appointed as his house surgeon in 1895. The technique of course relied on carbolic acid killing bacteria in the wound, which were being shed from the clothing of the surgical team and from surgical instruments all the time. Ogston's filthy operating coat, which was caked with dried blood, would have been hanging up in the operating theatre changing room ready to be put on and used for every case.

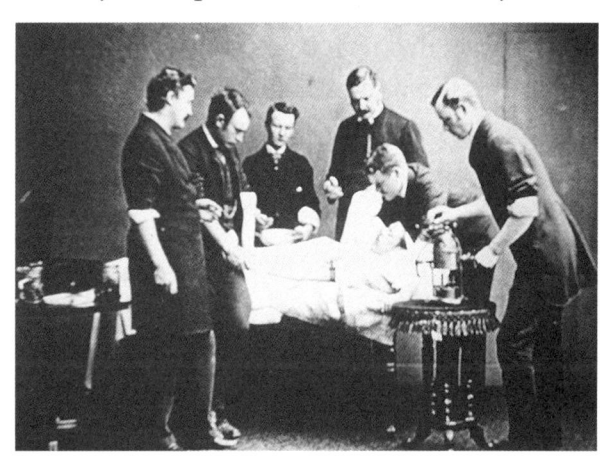

FIGURE 3.3

Sir Alexander Ogston at surgery illustrating antiseptic surgery; Ogston is on far left of the photograph. There is a carbolic dispenser on the far right to spray the wound and instruments with carbolic acid.

The Royal Army Medical Corps

Ogston was influential in helping to establish the Royal Army Medical Corps in 1898. He was one of a group of three prominent men who lobbied the Secretary of State for War, Lord Lansdowne. Sir Thomas Granger Stewart, President elect of the British Medical Association led the deputation. The third member of the group was Surgeon General Mouat VC, who had won his Victoria Cross in the

---

6   Scotland, T., and S. Heys, *Wars, Pestilence and the Surgeon's Blade*. Solihull: Helion and Co., 2013, p.303.

Crimean War, rescuing a wounded officer during the Charge of the Light Brigade at the battle of Balaclava in 1854. The three men successfully argued the case for improved conditions for medical officers in the army, without which it would never get good doctors, since no one would consider applying for a commission until medical officers were treated on an equal basis with any other officer.[7] Throughout the nineteenth century, army doctors had been regarded as neither officers nor gentlemen, as Gray's Uncle Robert would have known only too well.[8]

Gray makes a good impression with his teachers

During the year he spent as Ogston's house surgeon, Gray took every opportunity to gain as much experience as possible and played a very important role in looking after the patients in the ward.[9] It is documented that he took a greater interest than usual in the work of the 'dressers', a term which means surgical assistants. He received the following reference from Ogston after the completion of his house surgical post.

> University of Aberdeen
>
> 27 April, 1896
> Surgery Department
> Professor Alexander Ogston
>
> Although it will not be easy to do so, I am anxious adequately to express my sense of the work which MR HENRY M GRAY has done during the year just elapsed, during which he has had charge of my Department in the Aberdeen Royal Infirmary. I do not think such work as he has given could be surpassed by any one and this in every respect. More particularly, it is, I deem, a duty that I should specify

---

7 Cantlie, N., *A History of the Army Medical Department*. Edinburgh: Churchill Livingston, 1974, Volume 2, p. 359.
8 The reader will remember that Robert was an army surgeon in India in the 1860's.
9 Obituary, *British Medical Journal*, *op. cit.*, p. 814.

his kindness, attention, and humanity to all patients, and to the often troublesome but natural demands of their friends and those who correspond concerning them. The admirable and exhaustive diagnoses, reports and case taking he has carried out without failing in one single case to give every imaginable care and take every possible trouble; the minuteness, regularity and intelligence shown in the records he has kept; the unusual ability and skill he has exhibited in diagnoses; the perfection with which every preparation was made for all surgical operations and proceedings; the devotion expressed in the after-attention and dressing of the cases, whereby the mortality has been very notably diminished; and the knowledge and judgement displayed in his suggestions, often most valuable regarding the treatment of cases, have all strongly impressed me with a great respect for Mr Gray's ability as a Surgeon, and have persuaded me that he has, if ordinarily fortunate, a distinguished career ahead of him.

It has been a pleasure to work with Mr Gray, and I regret to part with one who, in addition to his brilliant qualifications, is a high principled and courteous member of our profession in a degree that is not often met with, I have had many admirable Resident Surgeons, but Mr Gray is the best of them I have ever had.

ALEX OGSTON

Gray also subsequently received a reference from Dr Matthew Hay, another very well known and distinguished Aberdeen doctor. Hay was Professor of Medical Logic and Jurisprudence (Forensic Medicine) at the University of Aberdeen, who also made many improvements in Public Health. Hay was influential in proposing what was called the Joint Hospital Scheme, where the Royal Infirmary, Maternity Hospital, Children's Hospital and Medical School in Aberdeen would all be built on the same site. Many years later on 6 February 1920, Hay chaired a preliminary meeting to put this into effect. One of the members of the committee was (the by then) Sir Henry Gray.[10]

---

10 Adam, A., J. Hutchison, *The Heritage of the Med-Chi, Aberdeen Medico-Chirurgical Society*. 2007, p. 54.

14, Rubislaw Terrace
Aberdeen, 6 January 1900

I have the fullest confidence in recommending Dr H.M.W. Gray for the assistant Surgeoncy of the Sick Children's Hospital. I know of no one within the city that possesses stronger qualifications for the post and the hospital is, in my opinion, in having within its offer the services of so able and competent a man. Gray is one of two or three men in the city, who are devoting themselves entirely to Surgery to the exclusion of other forms of medical practice, and is a specialist in that important and difficult branch of medicine. The claims of such men require the fullest consideration and sympathy when hospital posts in their special line of work fall vacant, especially when, in the case of Dr Gray, they are men of high ability and the requisite attitude and have for years been specially training themselves for these posts. I shall conclude by saying that it is a matter of common talk among the medical men of the city, that Dr Gray is one of the most promising young surgeons that our University has produced in recent years.

MATTHEW HAY
MD Honorary FRCPI
Professor of Forensic Medicine, University of Aberdeen; Medical Officer of Health
City of Aberdeen; President of the Society of Medical Officers of Health of Scotland[11]

Aseptic Surgery

As the germ theory of disease became more widely accepted, it was soon realised that infection could be better avoided by preventing bacteria from getting into wounds in the first place. While Lister and his contemporaries used antiseptics to destroy bacteria within wounds, they were still operating wearing filthy coats and tails and moving freely from one patient to the next in their blood-caked garments,

---

11 The references from Sir Alexander Ogston and Dr Matthew Hay come from the Gray Family Archives.

transferring bacteria as they went. If surgeons wore gowns which had been sterilised and if the surgical instruments they used were likewise sterilised and free from bacteria, then harmful organisms would have much less chance of gaining access to the wound.

Sterilisation of gowns and instruments

Ernst von Bergmann made a major breakthrough in aseptic surgery when he successfully sterilized surgical instruments by steam in 1885. Bergmann is also credited with using a similar method to sterilize wound dressings and other medical equipment used during surgical operations. Born in Latvia in 1836, Bergmann was Professor of Surgery at the Universities of Berlin and Wurzburg. Bergmann's method used steam under pressure and was the basis for modern sterilization procedures using autoclaves. Bergmann had previous experience of Lister's antiseptic surgical technique, having worked as a surgeon in the Franco-Prussian War (1870–71), when the Prussians used Lister's method.

Gray visits Germany

In 1896, after finishing his year as Ogston's Resident Surgeon, Gray went to Germany to complete his studies. The present day equivalent is a year spent as a 'fellow' towards the end of surgical training in a recognised centre of excellence, where some specific aspect of surgery of interest to the individual may be pursued at an advanced level. Gray spent a year and a half working in Bonn, Leipzig and Berlin, where he studied general surgery and gynaecology. He also developed a great interest in aseptic surgical techniques, which were far advanced in Germany. After spending some time in London on the way home, he was ready to introduce aseptic surgery to Aberdeen whenever the opportunity arose.[12]

Upon his return, he immediately started work as a surgeon

---

12 Obituary, Sir Henry Gray, KBE, FRCS, LLD, *The Lancet*, 15 October 1938, p. 920.

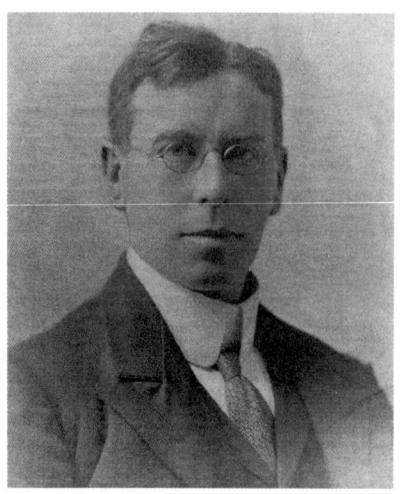

FIGURE 3.4
Henry Gray as a young man.

without any preliminary period in general practice, which was the usual thing to do at the time. Gray's atypical career pathway was resented by some prominent members of the medical profession and Gray had a difficult time to begin with. Never one for being diverted from his goal, Gray 'pursued the even tenor of his way'.[13]

Gray's appointments to Aberdeen Royal Infirmary

Gray became assistant anaesthetist to Aberdeen Royal Infirmary in 1897, which may well have been a 'filling in' post till the job he really wanted became vacant, because he became assistant surgeon the following year. To begin with, he had little opportunity to put any of his new ideas into practice. Like anyone working in post-graduate training, as an assistant surgeon he had to do what his 'chief' told him. He became a Fellow of the Royal College of Surgeons of Edinburgh in 1902. When Gray was appointed consultant surgeon to the Aberdeen Royal Infirmary in 1904 and became his own master, he could at last apply all his many ideas to clinical practice.

An interruption to surgical training: Gray's early military experience

Gray's surgical career was interrupted by the Second Boer War (1899–1902). While he would come to play a major role in delivering surgical care during the Great War (1914–18), he gained useful experience

---

13 Obituary, *British Medical Journal, op. cit.*, p. 814.

during this earlier conflict, when he served as a civilian surgeon in 1899 with Sir James Sievewright's Ambulance and was awarded the South African Medal with one clasp.[14] Gray was unfortunately invalided home with typhoid fever from South Africa. Sixty-four per cent of all deaths amongst British service personnel during the Second Boer War were caused by disease, mostly typhoid fever. Only thirty-six per cent of deaths were the result of enemy action. The cause of this high percentage mortality from disease was poor sanitation, allowing bacterial contamination of food and especially water supplies. In 1900, Gray was gazetted surgeon captain to the Aberdeen Volunteer Artillery and later was a major in the 1st Scottish General Hospital.[15]

Gray's Surgical Practice

After his appointment as Consultant Surgeon to Aberdeen Royal Infirmary, Gray worked extremely hard for the ten years before the outbreak of the Great War in August 1914. As well as introducing aseptic surgery, he is also credited with bringing local anaesthesia to surgery in Britain with Sir Herbert Barker of University College, London.[16]

Gray was truly a general surgeon. His lists might have a Caesarean section (then a very rare operation), an acute mastoid (a bone operation near the ear), a cerebral decompression (a brain operation), a hysterectomy (removal of womb), a total excision of urinary bladder and the plating of a fracture. Abdominal procedures were frequently done under spinal anaesthesia and operations on the limbs under local regional anaesthesia.[17]

Gray often operated on patients who had been turned down by other surgeons as a 'lost cause'. If a patient had received a verdict

---

14 Obituary, Sir Henry McIlree Williamson Gray, *Canadian Medical Association Journal*, Dec 1938, p. 612.
15 Obituary, *British Medical Journal*, *op. cit.*, p. 814.
16 Porter, R.M.M., *op. cit.*, pp. 11–13.
17 Porter, R.M.M., *op. cit.*, pp. 11–13.

elsewhere that it was too late, or that a condition was so far advanced as to be inoperable, Gray would assess the situation very carefully and offer the patient surgery if he thought there might be even a remote chance of success. Nowadays, as a result of close monitoring of surgeons' performances in league tables, many surgeons will shy away from difficult and risky procedures for fear of making their outcome statistics look unfavourable, resulting in censorship from hospital management. For those of Gray's patients who accepted the increased risk of surgery to get a chance to live, Gray used all his skill, technique, courage and patience to do his very best.[18] He always considered the patient first and if any criticism came his way when a risky procedure he had done failed, it didn't seem to affect him, outwardly at least.

Gray as a teacher

As a teacher, Gray was at his best at the bedside. There is evidence that he was not a good formal lecturer. The President of the Aberdeen Medico-Chirurgical Society, Dr Harold Edgar Smith said of him:

> In meetings of this Society, he was, shall I say, an indifferent speaker, but to me personally the tongue-tied hesitancy of his utterance, such was his personality, conveyed an honesty of purpose that eloquence often fails to achieve.[19]

By contrast, in the ward, if a student was enthusiastic and showed initiative, then Gray took endless pains to teach that individual. If any student suggested a particular course of action, then an understanding of how to put the suggested regime into practice would have to be displayed. On one occasion a student suggested that a turpentine enema would be a good solution for post operative flatulence. The pupil was told to go and administer it.[20] Surrounded by a dozen students in the ward and without a specific subject, Gray excelled. At

---

18 Obituary, *British Medical Journal, op. cit.*, p. 814.
19 Minutes of the Aberdeen Medico-Chirurgical Society. 27 October 1938.
20 Porter, R.M.M., *op. cit.,* pp. 11–13.

FIGURE 3.5

Old Aberdeen Royal Infirmary at Woolmanhill.

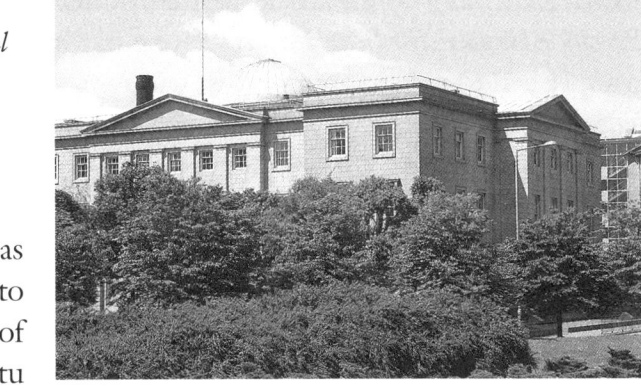

the time it was perhaps difficult to assess the value of these impromptu talks, but later on the recipients realised that their purpose was to make them think for themselves.[21]

Gray as consultant in charge of a team

Gray set himself very high standards, and there is certainly evidence in the literature that he expected the same from others, and was not easy to work for.

> His idealism in the surgical theatre was at times too high for the luckless assistant who fell short of expectation, and sharp reproof rang out in no uncertain way. It rankled at times, but geniality was resumed with the casting of the operating garment and the closing of the theatre door behind him.[22]

Another young house surgeon said of him:

> As a chief, he was sometimes very difficult. The good was never good enough. His language was often forceful and he did not tolerate fools gladly. No excuse was ever accepted for the shortcomings of the unfortunate house surgeon. Then his eyes would twinkle through his spectacles and a broad grin would spread over his face.[23]

---

21 Obituary, *The Lancet*, *op. cit.*, p. 920.
22 Obituary, *British Medical Journal*, *op. cit.*, p. 814.
23 Obituary *The Lancet*, *op. cit.*, p. 920.

In an addendum to an article written by R.M.M. Porter entitled *Recent Aberdeen Medical Teachers*,[24] one of Gray's former students who wished to remain anonymous, wrote:

> Of a surety one of the decisive days of my life was the day I first entered the ward of Mr. H.M.W. Gray as a dresser. Quickly he impressed on all his dressers the necessity of work, work, all the time, and scrupulous care in all we did, and all for the welfare of the patients committed to our care. What we had to do in the course of our duty just had to be done, and 'no time' was no excuse.

He continued:

> He was the first surgeon in Aberdeen to do a Caesarean section. He was well known in many distant lands: for example, he was visited when I was his house surgeon at Aberdeen Royal Infirmary by one of the brothers Mayo and while I was at the Children's Hospital by Von Perthes from Tubingen who came over to see him operate on inguinal hernia in infants, for he was one of the first to appreciate that all that was needed was to remove the sac (of the hernia) up to its neck.[25]

To be Gray's house surgeon was a highly sought after prize and even although the post was always hard and difficult, it was worth it, 'because to be trained by Gray gave young and up-coming surgeons confidence and standing that boded well for future success.'[26]

---

24 Porter, R.M.M., *op. cit.*, pp. 11–13.
25 William and Charles Mayo formed a surgical partnership from which evolved the cooperative group clinic, later known as the Mayo Clinic. Von Perthes too was a famous clinician who gave his name to Perthes' Disease, a disorder of the hip in childhood.
26 Smith, F.K., Sir Henry Gray, KBE, CB, CMG, *The Aberdeen University Review*, 1939, Vol XXVI, pp. 47–49.

FIGURE 3.6
Cartoon of Henry Gray.

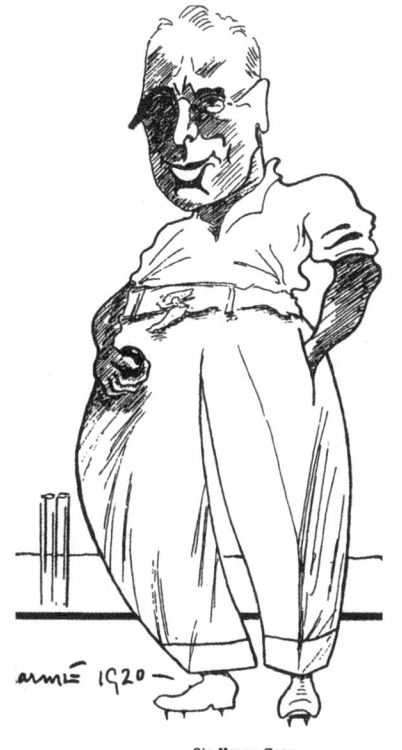

Sir Henry Gray

Gray applies unsuccessfully for the Chair of Surgery at the University of Aberdeen

Sir Alexander Ogston retired from the Professorship of Surgery in 1909. Gray had been a consultant for five years and felt he was ready to apply for the vacant Chair of Surgery. He wrote to his younger sister Eva:

> It is rather exciting this 'fecht'[27] for the Chair (of Surgery). It is curious the air of want of any intent in the business which the various prospective candidates show to the outside world, when I fancy there are all sort of plannings and plotting going on. I think on the whole that I shall get a lot of influence to bear . . .

Gray was unsuccessful in his application and the Professorship of Surgery went to John Marnoch, a lecturer in clinical surgery at the University of Aberdeen. Marnoch remained in post until 1932. When Gray returned to Aberdeen after the Great War, he would have realised there was no prospect of any academic progress, and this would have contributed to his decision to go to Montreal.

The Moynihan Provincial Surgical Club

Gray was no parochial surgeon. He believed in wide reading and made frequent visits to other surgeons, both at home and abroad.

---

27 A 'fecht' is a fight or a contest.

FIGURE 3.7
Sir Berkeley Moynihan.

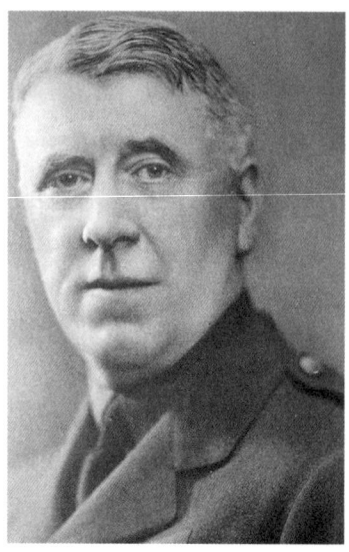

He was one of the original members of the Moynihan Provincial Surgical Club. Sir Berkeley Moynihan (1865–1936) was a powerful general surgeon from Leeds who set up this club in 1909 to bring together like-minded men in order to advance their surgical skills through visits to important clinics, while at the same time cementing professional and political ideals.[28] The formation of the club also demonstrated to the surgical establishment in London that surgical innovation could flourish out with the capital city. The first meeting was held on 23 July of that year. Seventeen surgeons from around the country went to the meeting, all hand-picked by Moynihan, who declared in an air of effortless superiority:

> I wish it to be clearly understood that I am not in competition with my London colleagues.[29]

Another surgeon who was invited by Moynihan to be a founding member of the Provincial Surgical Club and who subsequently became a good friend of Gray was Robert Jones (1857–1933) from Liverpool. Moynihan had the greatest respect for Jones, whom he referred to affectionately as 'Grandpa'. Moynihan once said 'No surgeon of international reputation smokes.'[30] Robert Jones at the time was almost a chain-smoker!

---

28 Cooter, R., *Surgery and Society in Peace and War*. Basingstoke: MacMillan Press Ltd., 1993, p.50.
29 Platt, H., 'Moynihan; The Education and Training of the Surgeon. Eleventh Moynihan Lecture delivered University of Leeds 25 May 1961', *Annals of the Royal College of Surgeons of England* 1962; 30: pp.220–228.
30 Platt, H., *op. cit.*

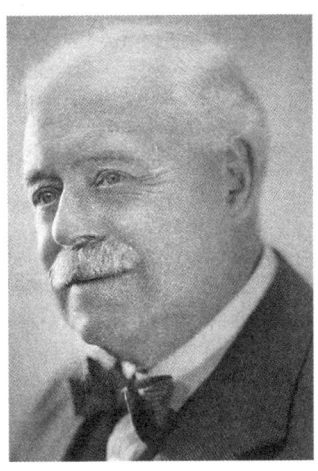

FIGURE 3.8
Sir Robert Jones.

Jones had acquired particular expertise in the management of musculoskeletal (orthopaedic) injuries. His interest in orthopaedics was initially stimulated by the work of his uncle by marriage, Hugh Owen Thomas (1834–1891), with whom he stayed from the age of sixteen. Thomas's clinical practice was in Nelson Street in Liverpool, close to the docks, where most of his patients lived in poverty. Many suffered from tuberculosis, which usually affected the lungs, but could also cause disease in bones and joints. Thomas was an eccentric medical practitioner, who was descended from a long line of 'bone setters'. Although he published his work, he never appended his medical qualifications, with the result that many thought that he, like his ancestors, was an unqualified 'bone setter.' Thomas never held a hospital appointment, but worked from his premises in Nelson Street. He invented many splints, including one to treat tuberculosis of the knee joint. Its purpose was to completely immobilise the joint in as good a position as possible, while the disease process inexorably destroyed the joint surfaces and ligaments before hopefully going on to partial healing by forming fibrous (scar) tissue. Such a destroyed joint would be stable in a reasonably good position, as opposed to being completely disorganised or even dislocated as a result of inadequate or no immobilisation. The Thomas Knee Splint would come to be used for immobilising and treating fractures of the femur (thigh bone) in the fullness of time and would assume a role of great importance during the First World War.

Inspired by his uncle, Jones studied medicine at the University of Liverpool and became a Fellow of the Royal College of Surgeons of Edinburgh. Unlike his uncle, Jones was outgoing and friendly and held a hospital appointment at the Southern General Hospital in Liverpool. He was appointed to the position of surgeon-superintendent during the construction of the Manchester Ship Canal between 1887 and 1894, when in strategically positioned hospitals he treated more than 3,000 injuries sustained by workers. He had to deal with 200 major injuries during this time including many affecting the musculoskeletal system.[31] No doubt, he found his uncle's Thomas Splint useful for treating fractures of the femur.

Jones' experience would stand him in good stead during the Great War, when orthopaedic wounds were extremely common. It would also bring him into a close working relationship with Henry Gray, who by then had developed a particular interest and expertise in the management of such wounds. By 1916, Gray had become the leading military orthopaedic surgical authority on the Western Front. Sir Berkeley Moynihan too would play a pivotal role in the development of orthopaedic surgery as will become clear. Indeed, the development of this speciality during the Great War owed a great deal to the Provincial Surgical Club, which became a major force to be reckoned with.

Gray's attitude to the wearing of gloves

The reader may be surprised by this sub-heading and wonder what bearing it has on the narrative. In the 21st Century, all surgeons wear disposable surgical gloves which have been sterilised by ionising radiation. It is routine practice to wear surgical gloves and there is nothing remarkable about it. Often gloves are changed during an operation, and once the procedure is finished, the gloves are disposed of. Furthermore, modern gloves are strong but very thin so that tactile sensation in the wound is unimpaired. This was not always the case. In 1909, Gray co-authored a book entitled *The practice of*

---

31 Watson, F., *The Life of Sir Robert Jones*. London: Hodder & Stoughton, 1934, p. 63.

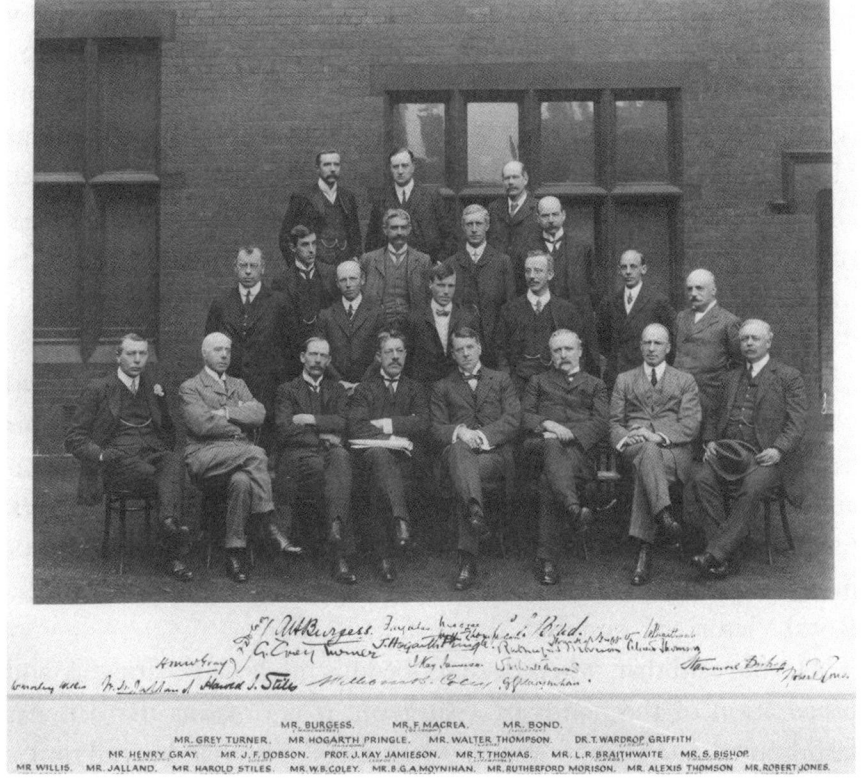

FIGURE 3.9

Moynihan Club Henry Gray 2nd row far left; Sir Berkeley Moynihan, centre front row; Robert Jones, front row far right.

anaesthetics and general surgical technique.[32] At the time he wrote this book, surgical gloves were in a relatively early stage of development. The first recorded instance of the wearing of gloves during an operation was in 1889, when one particularly good nurse at the Johns Hopkins Hospital in Baltimore found that constant washing of her hands and surgical instruments in carbolic acid was giving her severe dermatitis. To save her from having to continually expose her hands

---

32 Gray, H.M.W., with Collum, R.W., *The practice of anaesthetics and general surgical technique.* Edited by James Cantlie,. NY, 1909, W. Wood and Co., 396p.

to the acid, surgeon-in-chief, William Stewart Halsted designed and commissioned a rubber glove from the Goodyear Rubber Company. It must have been very inflexible compared with the modern version. Joseph Bloodgood, another of the surgeons at the Johns Hopkins Hospital and one of William Stewart Halsted's assistants, encouraged all members of the surgical team to wear newer-style, more flexible rubber gloves which had by then been developed. By the early 1900s, increasing numbers of surgeons and theatre nurses were routinely wearing surgical gloves.[33]

However, many surgeons in the early 20th Century still operated with bare hands. In the introduction to the surgical section of his book, Gray made it clear that he did not wear surgical gloves. This is an important point to emphasise, because as will be explained later, his aversion to wearing gloves would become a contributory factor in his downfall after he had been appointed Surgeon-in-Chief to the Royal Victoria Hospital in Montreal in 1923.

Having said that, when he described his methods for the care and preparation of the hands of a surgeon, it is obvious that he was fastidious about maintaining the cleanliness of his hands at all times. He believed that the disinfection of the hands immediately before performing an operation was of great importance, but he also believed that it was the duty of a surgeon to care for his hands at all times. He wrote:

> In addition, at all other times, it is of the greatest importance to keep the hands clean during every day activities. The surgeon should avoid handling anything which might soil his hands in a surgical sense. He should keep the hands smooth and well cared for. He should wear gloves constantly in winter when out of doors, during indulgence in field sports, pastimes, or gardening, otherwise his hands may become infected with organisms or spores which are particularly difficult to get rid of.[34]

---

33 http://www.ehow.com/about_6572251_history-surgical-gloves.html
34 Gray, H.M.W., with Collum, R.W., *op. cit.*, pp. 212–213.

In fact Gray had a pair of gloves for every occasion with the exception of the operating theatre. He went into great detail about how the hands and nails should be maintained and how Vaseline should be employed to prevent the skin drying up and cracking, particularly when using plaster of Paris. Bacteria should be removed from the hands by mechanical means (scrubbing in soap and water) before applying various antiseptic agents, after which 'the knocked-about, poison-soaked microbe has no chance in the warfare against the forces brought against it'. Gray conceded that bacteriologists maintained that it was quite impossible to make the hands sterile, but the best possible effort had to be made. Before the hands were thrust into the depth of the wound, they should be washed in sterile saline solution to remove bacteria inadvertently picked up from the skin. During a prolonged procedure, the hands should be treated several times in this way.

Gloves in the early and mid 20th Century

There were two types of surgical glove employed-rubber and cotton. Gray declared that their routine use by anyone made it appear that the user would not, or could not take proper care in the preparation of his hands. Cotton gloves were worn under the rubber gloves by some surgeons to stop moisture-bearing infected material building up beneath the rubber gloves, which would then pour into the wound should the glove be accidentally punctured. Unlike modern gloves, which are discarded after a single use, gloves during the early part of the century were re-used and sterilised by autoclaving or boiling. The orthopaedic co-author is very grateful to one of his senior former colleagues at Aberdeen Royal Infirmary, who was a student at the Westminster Hospital in London in 1951. The arrangement for the wearing of gloves in theatre was as follows. The consultant performing the operation wore a new pair gloves. The first assistant wore a pair that had been used once before, while the second assistant wore a pair which had been used twice. The student attached to the firm wore a pair that had been used three times. At night time, when things were quiet, the theatre staff detected leaks in the gloves which had been used that day by blowing into them and then repairing any holes by gluing on patches cut from gloves that were finished with and beyond repair, before boiling or autoclaving them, ready for use the next day. On one occasion the co-author's colleague inadvertently put on the 'chief's' new gloves, with dreadful consequences.

Gray stated that his results were no better when he wore gloves than when he did not.[35] He felt that gloves were a handicap to fine touch and manipulation. He could not palpate so well with gloves. He could not separate adhesions with the same assurance. He felt that gloves predisposed the surgeon to making too big an incision, a state of affairs he blamed von Bergmann for.

Gray felt strongly that students and other 'immature or inexperienced assistants' constituted an imminent danger to aseptic healing of the wound and should always wear gloves. The operator alone should put his bare hands in the depth of the wound, so that he alone was responsible for what occurred there.

He felt that the only good reason to wear gloves was for dealing with an infected case, when the main purpose of rubber gloves was to stop the hands of the surgeon becoming contaminated.

Gray's hospitality and other interests

Gray was an excellent host, and on Sunday evenings he often invited colleagues for supper to his home at 34 Albyn Place. He gathered together old and young, distinguished and undistinguished, and in the informal talks which followed the meal, Gray derived enormous pleasure hearing his house surgeon arguing with the most famous surgeons in the country.[36] Gray enjoyed Gilbert and Sullivan and would often block book seats to take members of his staff, both medical and nursing, to the theatre. Members of the D'Oyly Carte Opera Company often stayed with him at 34, Albyn Place.[37]

---

35 *Ibid.*, p. 222.
36 Obituary *The Lancet, op. cit.*, p. 920.
37 Porter, R.M.M., *op. cit.*, pp. 11–13.

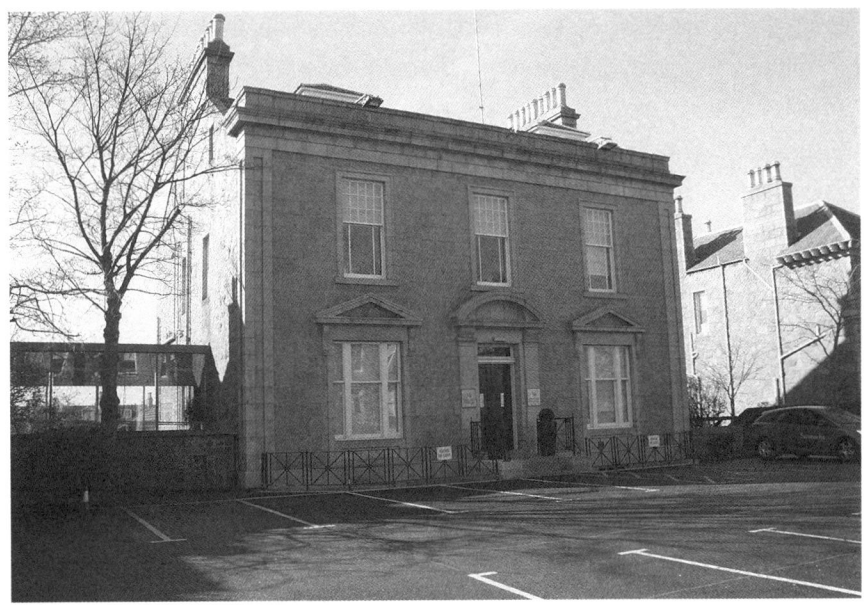

FIGURE 3.10
Gray's home 34 Albyn Place, Aberdeen.

Gray was a very keen cricketer, and played for Aberdeenshire for many years from 1889. His attendances at matches were somewhat inconsistent, which would have been the result of his clinical commitments. He was a good all rounder and was a very useful bowler. For example, in 1889,

> The first match of the season was against Orion who, thanks to the fine bowling of H.M.W. Gray, (six, all bowled, for 9) were dismissed for 33.

It was through the Aberdeenshire Cricket Club that he knew his colleague John Christie who enrolled at Medical School the same time as Gray. Christie went on to become a dermatologist and in 1903 was put in charge of skin diseases at Aberdeen Royal Infirmary – first as Assistant Physician and then in 1910 as Full Physician.

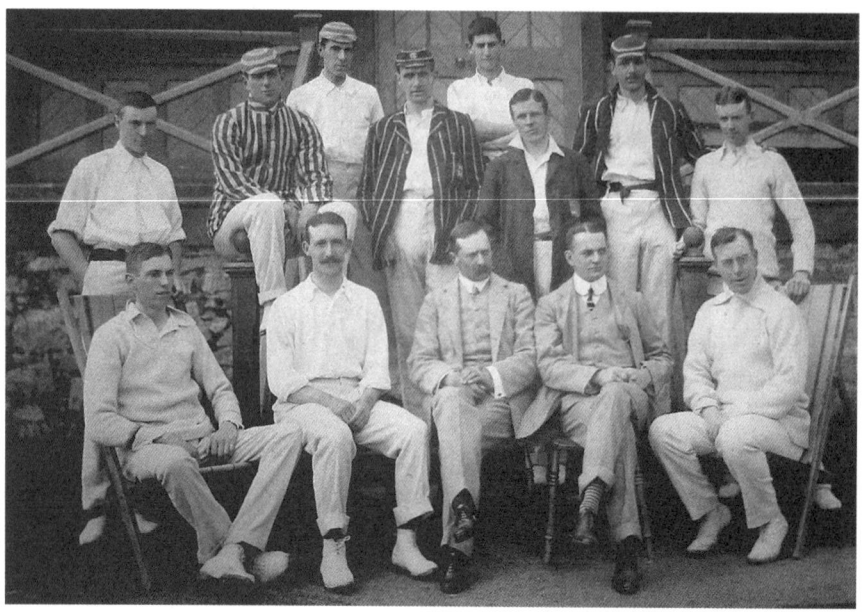

FIGURE 3.11

Gray in photograph Aberdeenshire Cricket Club; Gray front row, far right.

This completes the account of the first phase of Gray's surgical career. As a trainee, he had obviously made a very good impression, while as a consultant he was a brave clinician who dealt with many difficult cases which others surgeons steered clear of. His enormous clinical experience and expertise would stand him in very good stead for the second phase of his career which began in August 1914 with the outbreak of the First World War.

CHAPTER 4

Gray's career during the Great War

At the outbreak of the Great War in August 1914, Henry Gray immediately volunteered his services to treat the wounded and joined the Royal Army Medical Corps with the rank of temporary major. At first he was seconded to a Red Cross Unit at Wimeraux, but finding insufficient scope for his surgical skills, he returned briefly to Britain before going back to France, where he spent the next three and a half years, at first in charge of a group of base hospitals in Rouen and then consulting surgeon to the British Third Army. His task was to ensure that soldiers who had sustained appalling wounds received the best possible surgical care, and Gray became one of the most outstanding consulting surgeons in France. He was a 'hands-on' clinician and remained so throughout the conflict. He was greatly admired by the young surgeons working under his supervision to whom he gave every support. His skills and expertise were second to none and were widely acknowledged and appreciated, not just by the British Third Army for which he was directly responsible, but by the other four British Armies too. His achievements are reflected in his service record, summarised here in the University Of Aberdeen Roll Of Service in The Great War.

- Major, R.A.M.C.(T), 1914. Seconded for service with British Hospital (Red Cross) at Wimereux;
- Nov. 1914. Col., A.M.S., Consultant Surg., BEF, Feb 1915;
- Consultant, Special Mil. Surgery (Home Service) June 1918;
- Served France, Nov. 1914-June 1918; Home, June 1918-June 1919. Final Rank, Colonel;
- K.B.E.(mil), C.B.(mil), C.M.G.(mil). Five mentions.[1]

---

1 University of Aberdeen, Roll of Service in the Great War 1914–1919. Edited by M.D. Allardyce, Aberdeen University Press. 1921.

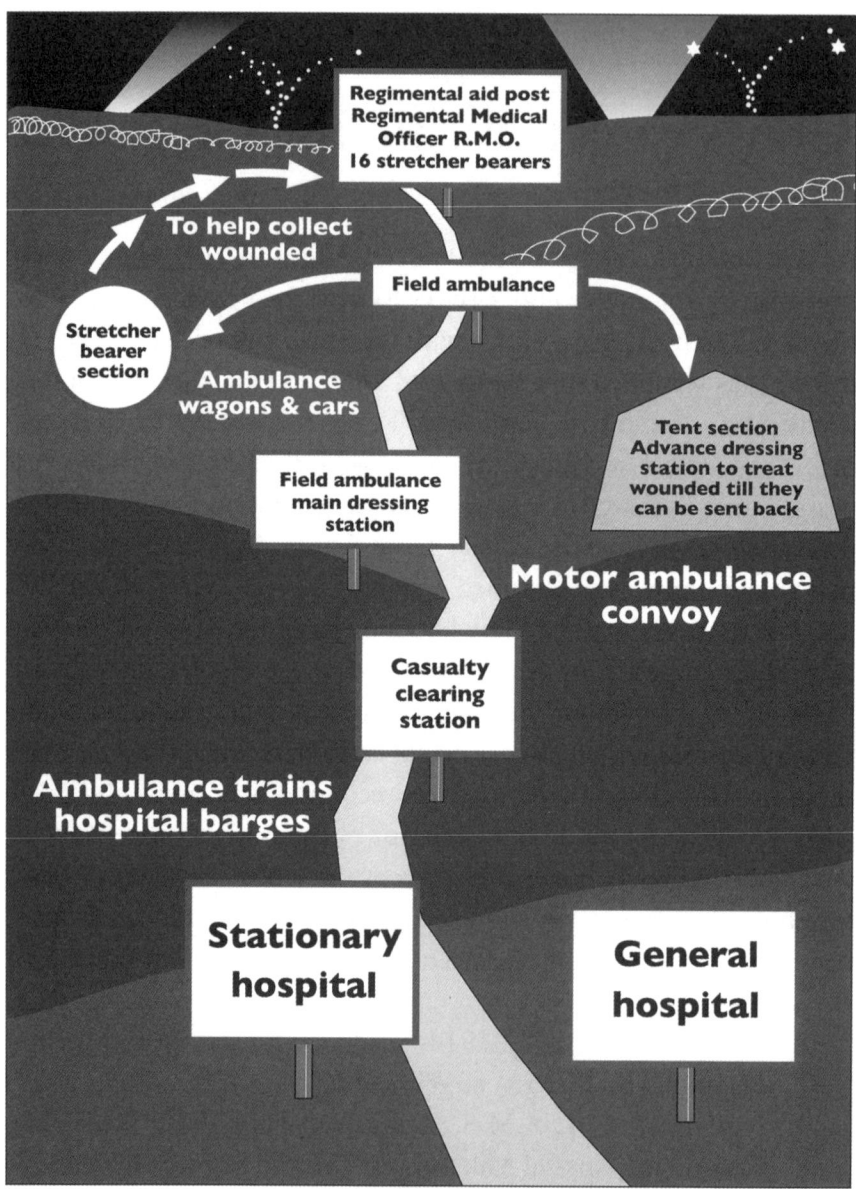

FIGURE 4.1
Evacuation pathway for the wounded.

Gray's contribution to the advance of surgery during the Great War earned him a knighthood and subsequently an Honorary Degree of LLD from the University of Aberdeen in 1924.[2]

The evacuation pathway for the wounded from the Western Front

It is important to understand the evacuation pathway for the wounded and how it evolved in response to huge numbers of casualties with filthy contaminated wounds, the likes of which had never been seen by the attending surgeons before. Each battalion of approximately 1,000 officers and men had a regimental medical officer (RMO) who was responsible for treating the sick and wounded. The RMO had sixteen regimental stretcher bearers (increased to 32 during a major attack) whose job it was to retrieve the wounded from No Man's Land and transport them to the Regimental Aid Post close to the front line, where they were given basic first aid before a field ambulance took over their care. A field ambulance was a mobile medical facility positioned quite close to the front line. Each ambulance had 10 officers and 224 men, who worked in either a tent division or a stretcher bearer division, to serve a brigade of approximately 4,000 infantrymen. Each ambulance was subdivided into three identical sections, lettered A, B or C, and theoretically capable of independent action. In practice, the sections worked closely together, since the front line was static for most of the war and scarcely moved at all. Consequently there was no need for independent action. Three field ambulances were allocated to an infantry division of three brigades (approximately 12,000 men). The tent divisions of the ambulances were responsible for establishing a divisional advanced dressing station (ADS) approximately two miles from the front line and a main dressing station (MDS) a further two miles to the rear. The ADS and MDS were treatment facilities for the wounded. The stretcher bearer divisions of the ambulances combined

---

2 The Aberdeen University Review. 1923–24; XI: p. 272.

resources to collect the wounded from Regimental Aid Posts and take them to the ADS or MDS. Surgery was rarely performed at ADSs during the early years of the conflict, although by 1918 the re-establishment of mobile warfare resulted in the development of field ambulance resuscitation teams by personnel from the five Australian Divisions, when experienced surgeons, who were capable of performing limb and life-saving surgery, went forward to operate on badly wounded soldiers in advanced dressing stations. More will be said about field ambulance resuscitation teams later in the chapter. From the ADS, patients were transported to the MDS or to clearing hospitals, depending on the severity of their wounds. Clearing hospitals were renamed casualty clearing stations (CCSs) in 1915. The personnel at a casualty clearing station comprised eight officers and seventy-seven other ranks. One medical officer had dental qualifications. Nursing sisters were introduced in 1915, at first five and then seven. Casualty clearing stations were usually out of range of shell fire, at a minimum of 10,000 yards from the front line and could be reached relatively quickly by motor ambulance wagon convoys from advanced dressing stations. They were usually constructed from pre-fabricated wooden huts in close proximity to a railway line. Each had accommodation for approximately 800–1,200 wounded. Their initial purpose in 1914 was to clear casualties by hospital train to base hospitals for definitive surgery, but this took too long and resulted in many unnecessary deaths from overwhelming infection secondary to delay in effective surgical management. Patients with filthy contaminated wounds needed definitive surgical treatment as soon as possible after the infliction of the wound and it was necessary to operate on such patients before they were sent by train to the base. Medical and nursing staff experienced in the treatment of soldiers with limb and life threatening wounds were sent to casualty clearing stations where this work was undertaken. A casualty clearing station normally had two surgical teams during 'quiet' spells, each consisting of a surgeon, anaesthetist, theatre sister and an operating theatre orderly. When reinforcements were required during a battle, surgical teams were sent from tent sections of field ambulances, from other CCSs in quiet sectors and from base hospitals.

Gray as Consulting surgeon to base hospitals in Rouen

Gray became consulting surgeon to a group of base hospitals in Rouen in February 1915. In February 1916 he had the opportunity to pay a visit to the British medical facilities in the army areas on the Western Front. He wrote to Eva:

> I have just come back from a most interesting, instructive and sometimes dangerous trip round our three armies here.[3] I found that things were extraordinarily good in arrangements for sick and wounded and preventive treatment. Quite proud to belong to the Corps[4] temporarily; they have done well in this great show. I was in time for the fight on 11th and following days on the Ypres Salient.[5] Travelled through Poperinghe and Vlamertinghe[6] etc. on the Salient, but was not allowed into Ypres-too hot to ask such an important passenger-Haw! Haw! Had aeroplanes overhead dropping bombs; was in the trenches in Givenchy and had a squint over the parapet at the Germans as well as through a periscope. Know what it is like to be under shrapnel, shell and rifle fire and was jolly glad to get out of it too. Windy Corner,[7] where I started from is reported to be quite an unhealthy spot, but things were I should say fairly quiet really. They

---

3 By later in 1916 there would be five British Armies in France and Flanders
4 The medical facilities for which the Corps or Armies were responsible were the facilities close to the front line-the regimental aid posts, field ambulances and casualty clearing stations. Gray at the time was attached to base hospitals on the lines of communication.
5 There were German operations in the area of the Bluff on the southern part of Ypres Salient which lasted for a few days till noon on 17 February 1916 and cost the British 1,294 casualties.
6 Poperinghe and Vlamertinghe were places to the west of Ypres. There was a main dressing station at Vlamertinghe and casualty clearing stations at Poperinghe.
7 Windy corner was a cross-road between Bethune and la Bassée close to the village of Cuinchy.

(the Germans) plonked a shell into a dugout regimental aid post a short time after I was there and killed some men. I liked the snipers' bullets worst of all-one could hear them smack occasionally-too near for 'Lil Gray's' taste, although he did keep his head well down!

In June 1915, a paper was published in the British Medical Journal which explained how the medical arrangements at the base hospitals in Rouen worked and mentioned Gray by name.[8] Here is a précis of these arrangements, described by the 'special correspondent in France' who wrote the paper. The hospitals utilised every available space including abandoned hospital buildings, schools and residential colleges, as well as specially constructed pine-huts for use as temporary hospital wards in which to carry out the work. Gray was in overall charge of surgical activity in these various hospitals and was head of a team which advised from time to time on what line of surgical treatment should be used for different types of wound. Surgeons with responsibility for the individual hospitals then put these recommendations into practice to give any proposed new treatment a fair trial. The work at the hospitals was extremely demanding and patients required all the skill and expertise which could be brought to bear to deal with dreadful wounds. Some of the cases are described in the paper.

- Abdominal wall torn by shell fragment with protrusion of intestines; small bowel resection and anastomosis (damaged bowel removed and the ends joined up) performed; patient survived;
- Shell wound cervical spine; patient quadriplegic (paralysis of all four limbs); shell splinter removed; neurological signs improved (the patient began to recover some function of his arms and legs);
- Fistula (abnormal communication) between subclavian artery

---

8 The War Medical Arrangements of the British Expeditionary Force. From a Special Correspondent in France. *British Medical Journal*, 12 June 1915; pp. 1020–1.

and vein (major vessels in the root of the neck and surgically difficult to gain access to) caused by bullet; no operative intervention at time of writing;
- Huge wound over spine with much muscle loss and dreadful tissue contamination; dead tissue excised;

Filthy, contaminated wounds in 1914
The accepted surgical practices in 1914 were based on experience derived from the Second Boer War (1899–1902) and were completely ineffective against multiple extensive wounds caused by fragments of shell casing and machine gun bullets which were characteristic of wounds sustained during the Great War. Such high energy wounds were associated with a great deal of tissue destruction, and huge amounts of dead muscle were contaminated by shell fragments and soil from the richly fertilised fields of France and Flanders. Wounded soldiers were evacuated to base hospitals for definitive surgery, and most patients reached these facilities with established major wound infections caused by staphylococci or streptococci. Many were suffering from gas gangrene, caused by the organism clostridium perfringens. Gangrene spreads rapidly along muscle fibres producing further muscle destruction and gas bubbles within the tissues, which imparts a crackling sensation on palpation of the affected extremity, hence the name gas gangrene. The release of a powerful toxin soon results in multiple organ failure and death. Clostridium perfringens is an anaerobic organism, which means it only grows in the absence of oxygen and wounds with a great deal of dead muscle, especially those of the thigh and buttock, were particularly susceptible.

Disastrous management of wounds in the early months of the war
During the first few months of the war, both in field ambulances and in the 'clearing hospitals,' wounds were superficially disinfected and sutured. This was hopelessly inadequate treatment. More effective surgical management at base hospitals could be delayed for several

days and the results were appalling. There is a statement in the Official Australian Medical History of the Great War which sums things up.

> During the first six months of the conflict the mortality and morbidity from 'septic' infection dealt to the surgical profession in every nation concerned a staggering blow, from which it recovered only through tedious and painful apprenticeship.[9]

Wound excision

New and more effective surgical methods had to be found, and Henry Gray led the way when he pioneered a procedure known as wound excision. This means the removal of *all* dead and contaminated tissue from the wound. It was a procedure which had to be performed early, before infection became established. Wound excision is a systematic procedure, excising dead skin, dead fat, dead and contused (bruised and/or crushed) underlying muscle and where there are fractures, removing debris and loose pieces of bone which have lost normal soft tissue attachments, before thoroughly cleansing and irrigating the tissues. Even apparently minor looking missile wounds might be grossly contaminated on the inside of the body from shell fragments carried into the depths of the wound. Unless all dead and contaminated tissue was completely excised, and unless there was nothing left but healthy, bleeding tissue, the operation would fail, with potentially catastrophic consequences for the patient. Under such circumstances, gas gangrene could become established and result in the loss of a soldier's limb or his life. In the early months of the war, many patients arrived at base hospitals in Rouen with established gangrene. As 1915 progressed, casualty clearing stations began to provide the essential facilities and resources for early wound excision, before the patient was sent by hospital train to the base hospitals. It was in large part

---

9 Butler, A.G., *Official History of the Australian Army Medical Services, 1914–1918 Volume II – The Western Front*. Canberra: Australian War Memorial, 1940, p. 312.

due to Gray's pioneering work that definitive surgery was performed at casualty clearing stations closer to the front.

First accounts of wound excision

The first published accounts of deliberate wound excision were described independently by Henry Gray and by E.T.C. Milligan. Gray as already stated, was working in hospitals in Rouen, while the latter, an Australian, was based in a casualty clearing station closer to the front line.[10] Milligan was a graduate of Melbourne University, who at the outbreak of war was engaged in special study in England and joined the RAMC. He published his work *The Early Treatment of Projectile Wounds by Excision of the Damaged Tissues*[11] in June 1915, while Gray published his paper in the Journal of the Royal Army Medical Corps the same month and went even further by proposing excision and primary closure of selected wounds.[12]

Gray also published his work in the British Medical Journal in August 1915 to make the method more widely known and understood.[13] He first began employing the technique of wound excision and primary closure in November 1914. To be successful, surgery had to be undertaken early, before the wound began to display the signs of infection with induration (a woody hardening) and erythema (redness) of the surrounding skin. The procedure involved the excision of all devitalised tissue, followed by suturing of the wound, allowing healing by first intention, which saved a great deal of time. Wounds treated this way required much less nursing care, pain was diminished, the number of dressings was reduced and complications of a septic wound were avoided. However, it was absolutely essential

---

10 Butler, *op. cit. p.* 326.
11 Milligan, E.T.C., The early treatment of projectile wounds by excision of the damaged tissue. *British Medical Journal* 1915; 1: p.1081.
12 Gray, H.M.W., The treatment of gunshot wounds by excision and primary suture. *Journal Royal Army Medical Corps* June 1915.
13 Gray, H.M.W., Treatment of Gunshot wounds by excision and primary suture. *British Medical Journal* 1915; 2: p. 317.

that *all* devitalised tissue was removed, otherwise wound closure over residual dead or contaminated tissue would inevitably result in major sepsis with the added risk of gas gangrene. The operation had to be performed by a sufficiently experienced surgeon exercising sound clinical judgement. Sometimes Gray might not have been sure of the completeness of a wound excision. Under such circumstances, he would leave the wound open and have a second look after 48 hours, when it was usually possible to close the wound if it looked healthy. This is called delayed primary closure. Sometimes the patient already had established infection when first operated upon, in which case dead and contaminated tissue was surgically removed from the wound and the wound left open for 12–14 days, before being closed by secondary suture. Antiseptic agents had a role to play in this situation. Sometimes the damage to tissues was so great that in the case of an arm or leg, primary amputation was the only safe course of action.

The place of antiseptics in the management of wounds

Much attention was given to the use of a wide variety of antiseptics, in an attempt to kill bacteria within wounds, while hopefully avoiding too much direct damage caused by the antiseptic to the surrounding healthy tissues. These methods included the use of salt packs, Bismuth, Iodine, Dakin's Solution (active ingredient sodium hypochlorite), Eusol (active ingredient chlorinated lime and boric acid), hydrogen peroxide and acriflavine, to give but a few examples.

It has been suggested that a technique developed by Alexis Carrel,[14] employing irrigation tubes to reach the depths of a wound and using Dakin's Solution as a germicide, was the main reason for reduction

---

14 Alexis Carrel was a distinguished French surgeon who did pioneering work before the war on stitching damaged blood vessels back together and was awarded a Nobel Prize for Medicine in 1912. Henry Dakin was an English chemist. The two men collaborated during the war and by employing a system of irrigation tubes, inserted deep into the recesses of a wound, delivered high concentrations on antiseptic agent to the depth of the wound.

in mortality of certain wounds, specifically compound fractures of the femur.[15] This is a complete misperception and it is important to realise that while antiseptic agents were used extensively, their use was no substitute for adequate surgery. Henry Gray wrote:

> It cannot be emphasised too urgently that the use of antiseptics will not make up for inadequate operative treatment. It can safely also be said that the stronger the antiseptic, the worse the result. The fact should be remembered when a particularly soiled wound tempts the use of strong remedies, or when one vaunted antiseptic is tested against another. On the other hand, provided the operation is adequate, one kind of rational after-treatment does not seem to influence the patient's chance of life or limb more than another.[16]

The Official History of the Australian Army Medical Services states:

> In practically all severe wounds admitted to C.C.S.s, it is found necessary to give anaesthetics to enable the damaged muscle, fascia, etc, bordering on the wound to be excised and foreign bodies removed, and to enable the surgeon to provide sufficient drainage. This is a preliminary to any form of treatment whether by 'Carrel,' salt pack or any other method of dressing. It is this measure alone which diminishes the danger of severe anaerobic infection.[17]

Gray's steadfast support of young surgeons

Gray was extremely supportive of Milligan, as he was of other young surgeons with whom he had the pleasure and privilege of working. For example in 1918, Surgeon-General Sir Anthony Bowlby delivered a paper on the excision and primary suture of wounds,

---

15 Cooter, R., *Surgery and Society in Peace and War*. Basingstoke: MacMillan Press Ltd, 1993, p. 111.
16 Gray, H.M.W., *The Early Treatment of War Wounds*. London: Henry Frowde and Hodder & Stoughton, 1919, p.107.
17 Butler, A.G., *op. cit.*, p. 329.

published in the British Medical Journal on 23 March 1918.[18] Bowlby made no mention of Milligan in his article, despite the fact that Milligan and Gray had independently been the first to describe the technique. Gray came swiftly to the aid of Milligan and other young surgeons who had been involved in the pioneering work. In the correspondence section of the British Medical Journal the following month he said:

> I feel it is only just, considering the knowledge of the facts which I possess, that credit and prominence should be given to the work of surgeons like Milligan, Charles, Lockwood, Roberts, Tabineau and the Andersons, who in 1914 and 1915 were laying the foundation, in an unostentatious way, of the recent work of which Sir Anthony writes. I am sure that the surgeons quoted in Sir Anthony Bowlby's paper would not wish that mention should be made of them alone.[19]

Gray continued:

> Many of the names I have mentioned above are attached to articles describing work and results of the excellence of which, in the early years of the war, was realised only by those who experienced them.[20]

Gray's meaning is clear. As well as being very supportive of enterprising young surgeons working under his leadership and instruction, he is sniping at Sir Anthony Bowlby, very much an establishment figure. Gray frequently did not get on with the 'surgical establishment,' epitomised by Bowlby. There are other examples of clashes between the two men in the medical literature and perhaps Gray would have been better to exercise diplomacy and self restraint. This might have helped to avoid future difficulties in his career, as will be explained later.

---

18 Bowlby, A., Primary suture of wounds at the front in France. *British Medical Journal* March 23, 1918, pp. 333–337.
19 Gray, H.M.W., Correspondence; Primary suture of war wounds. *British Medical Journal,* 20 April 1918, p. 467.
20 *Ibid.*

Management of fractures and the importance of the Provincial Surgical Club

The origin and aims of the Moynihan Provincial Surgical Club have already been discussed. Members of the Surgical Club would play very important roles during the Great War, helping to establish orthopaedics at the forefront of war surgery. In 1914, Robert Jones inspected the hospitals of Western Command as one of his wartime duties. He drew attention to large numbers of soldiers with fractures, whose initial management had been poor and who would require prolonged treatment in specialised orthopaedic units.[21] These men had often been passed from one hospital to another in order to free up beds and had not been provided with the necessary continuity of care to ensure the best possible outcome for their wounds. As a result, hospitals were full to overflowing with crippled soldiers, who were neither fit for military duty, nor for discharge back into civilian life. At the conclusion of his inspection, Jones wrote a damning report, which soon reached Sir Alfred Keogh, Director General of Army Medical Services.

In December 1914, Sir Berkeley Moynihan inspected hospitals in France. His visit lasted until March 1915, after which he was called upon by Sir Alfred Keogh. In providing Keogh with a summary of his visit to the medical facilities dealing with casualties from the Western Front, Moynihan expressed the view that the treatment of compound fractures in France was deplorable and that the country would soon be 'flooded by men doomed to deformity and crippling.'[22]

Sir Alfred Keogh authorised Jones to open an experimental orthopaedic unit with 250 beds (quickly becoming 560 beds) at Alder Hey Hospital in Liverpool in the spring of 1915, segregating patients with orthopaedic wounds for the first time. This was so

---

21 Watson, F., *The Life of Sir Robert Jones*. London: Hodder & Stoughton, 1934, p.147.
22 Platt, H., 'Moynihan; The Education and Training of the Surgeon. Eleventh Moynihan Lecture delivered University of Leeds 25 May 1961', *Annals of the Royal College of Surgeons of England* 1962; 30: pp.220–228.

successful that Jones became responsible for the first of many orthopaedic centres in March 1916. This centre was opened on the site of the Hammersmith Workshop in Shepherd's Bush in London. Amongst those he took advice from before setting it up was his good friend Henry Gray.[23] They concluded that a clearing house scheme offered the least objection and would invite least friction from the surgical establishment. Jones wrote:

> A clear definition of the scope covered by the term orthopaedics should be supplied to the CO of each general hospital in the Command, making him responsible for evacuation of orthopaedic cases from his hospital and its auxiliaries into a clearing house, to which should be attached a good surgeon of orthopaedic training.[24]

The orthopaedic centre at Shepherd's Bush was established in the back yard of the London surgeons and would be sure to cause resentment. Jones was basically saying that general hospitals were not competent to deal with a large percentage of the wounded. Shepherd's Bush fulfilled two important functions. Firstly, it provided surgical expertise to deal with late orthopaedic problems such non-union or mal-union[25] of fractures. Secondly, it provided a restorative workshop, which gave the recovering soldiers an occupation. For example, in an orthopaedic centre opened some time later in Aberdeen at the 1st Scottish General Hospital at Old Mill Hospital, better known today as Glenburn Wing, Woodend Hospital, one of the jobs soldiers did (in the workshop) was to mend nets for the deep sea fishing industry. This helped to restore the function of their arms and hands, while at the same time it improved morale by giving them something useful to do. For practical purposes, this was the start of what we call

---

23 Watson, F., *op. cit.*, p.165.
24 *Ibid.*
25 Non-union of a fracture means that the normal healing processes have failed and the fracture fails to unite. Infection is the usual cause. Mal-union means the fracture has united, but in a bad position resulting in a significant impairment in function.

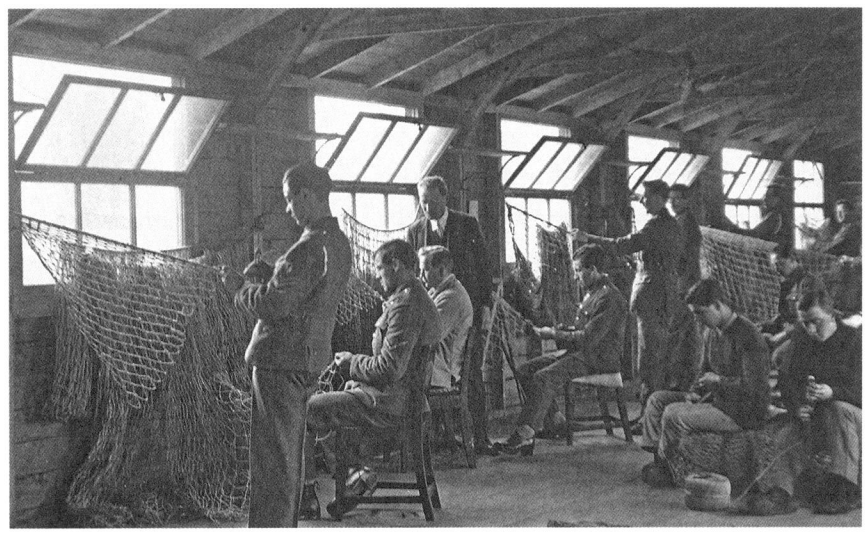

FIGURE 4.2
Soldiers in Oldmill Hospital, mending fishing nets in the restorative workshop.

occupational therapy today. A contract with the fishing industry also helped to pay for the centre.

At around the same time that Shepherd's Bush opened, Moynihan told Keogh that a Director of Military Orthopaedic Surgery was needed. Realising that Moynihan wanted Jones for the position, Keogh responded by saying that if he appointed Jones the London surgeons would have his head on a charger, to which Moynihan retorted that if Jones was not appointed, then he, Moynihan, would resign. So Jones became Director of Military Orthopaedics.

The emergence of orthopaedic surgery as a specialty did not please London establishment figures, who tried unsuccessfully to have Jones removed from office in 1916, when a formal objection to Jones' appointment was lodged with the President of the Royal College of Surgeons of England. Delivering the Eleventh Moynihan Lecture in Leeds on 25 May 1961, orthopaedic surgeon Sir Harry Platt described how Moynihan

... used all the eloquence at his command to dissuade the Council from taking a disastrous action. The College acted wisely.[26]

Moynihan was powerful enough to keep the London establishment under control, allowing Jones to use his energies to open orthopaedic centres round Britain in Manchester, Leeds, Newcastle, Oxford, Reading, Cardiff, Birmingham, Bristol, Bath, Dublin, Belfast, Edinburgh, Glasgow and Aberdeen.[27]

The College launched another major assault in 1918, when after a meeting of the council, chaired by its President, Sir George Makins, the following statement was made:

> It (the Council) regarded with mistrust and disapprobation the movement in progress to remove the treatment of conditions always properly regarded as the main portion of the general surgeon's work from his hands, and place it in those of 'orthopaedic surgeons' . . . And thus to educate the layman to the belief that the British surgeon is incapable of dealing with the majority of the most serious injuries the body may sustain.
>
> Minutes of Council, Royal College of Surgeons England, 16 July 1918[28]

Once again they were unsuccessful, although after the war was over, orthopaedics receded into the shadows for many years. Robert Jones had hoped that orthopaedic departments would be attached to every major hospital, but alas it wasn't to be. Symbolic of the prevailing mood, Shepherd's Bush was returned to its original function as a poor law infirmary and workhouse and most other orthopaedic centres met the same fate.

---

26 Platt, H., *op. cit.*, p.223.
27 Watson, F., *op. cit.*, p.181.
28 Cooter, R., *op. cit.*, p. 133.

Gray's contribution to acute orthopaedic services

By 1916, Gray was a leading authority in the management of compound gunshot fractures, particularly those of the femur.[29] In the official New Zealand medical history of the Great War, Lieutenant Colonel A D Carberry stated:

> Surgery, especially that of the front line, was a specialty of the Third Army whose Consulting Surgeon, Colonel H.M.W. Gray, was noted since 1916 for his work in the treatment of compound gunshot fractures. His memoranda, issued by the Third Army in 1917, formed the basis of the front line surgical practice of this and other armies. His well-known book, *The Early Treatment of War Wounds*, published at the end of 1918, epitomised the advancing knowledge of that period. His lectures given at Louvencourt were attended by all our medical officers in turn: the problems of shock prevention at the RAP and ADS, the best method of splinting fractures and the demonstration of the regulation set of splints now carried in racks by each motor ambulance, formed the basis of these lectures.[30]

Fractures of the femur

Compound fractures of the femur (thigh bone) were particularly serious because of the large amount of muscle damage sustained and the loss of at least a couple of pints of blood into the thigh. The huge area of the wound with many possible recesses predisposed to foreign bodies lying undetected within its depths. Pieces of shrapnel and contaminated clothing created the ideal setting for the establishment of major wound infection. Frequently the muscle had been so badly damaged that there were areas deprived of a blood supply and therefore of oxygen, giving the bacteria responsible for gas gangrene an opportunity to thrive.

Gray documented a mortality of around 80 per cent for compound

---

29 Gray, H.M.W., *The Early Treatment of War Wounds*. London: Henry Frowde and Hodder & Stoughton, 1919, pp. 59–60.
30 Carberry, A.D., *The New Zealand Medical Services in the Great War*. Auckland: Whitcombe and Tombs Ltd, 1924, p. 399.

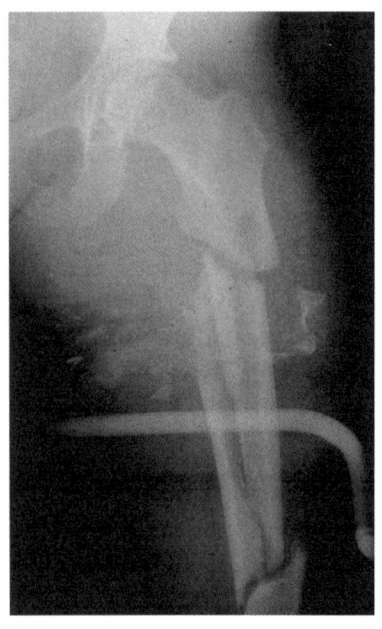

FIGURE 4.3
Fractured femur.

fractures of the femur in 1914 and early 1915, when splints employed to immobilise the broken bones were not fit for purpose and when there was significant delay in performing definitive surgery.[31] The only splint mentioned for dealing with fractures of the femur in the Royal Army Medical Corps Handbook of 1911 was the Rifle Splint, which failed to immobilise the fracture, resulting in uncontrolled movement of the broken bone ends during transport of the patient and excessive blood loss. Consequently, patients arrived at casualty clearing stations in hypovolaemic shock (shock due to severe loss of blood).

Robert Jones made a very important contribution to acute orthopaedic services on the Western Front. With the encouragement of Gray, he introduced the Thomas Splint to deal with fractures of the femur. The Thomas Splint immobilised the fracture much more effectively, restricting movement at the fracture site and reducing bleeding, so that patients arrived at casualty clearing stations in good

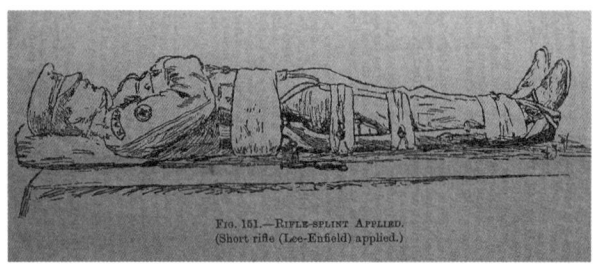

FIGURE 4.4
Rifle Splint.

---

31 Gray, H.M.W., *The Early Treatment of War Wounds*. London: Henry Frowde and Hodder & Stoughton, 1919, p. 59.

FIGURE 4.5
Thomas Splint.

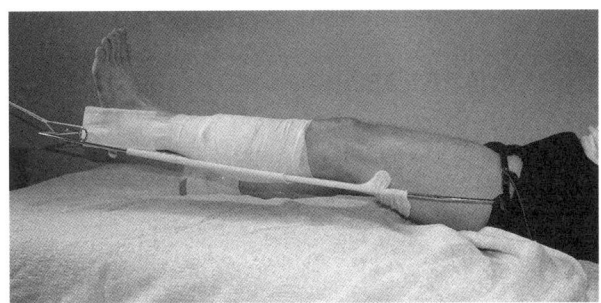

clinical condition and fit to undergo wound excision. The top of the splint fitted snugly against the pelvis and groin area while the leg rested on canvas slings. Skin traction was then applied and cords at the bottom of the traction system were pulled on very firmly to get the fractured bone ends out to length and into good position. This also had the effect of stretching the muscles of the thigh, overcoming muscle spasm and relieving pain.[32] The cords were then tied round the bottom of the splint, making sure that a good steady pull was maintained to hold the fracture in good position. The casualty could then be transported relatively easily and with little pain from the front line to casualty clearing stations specialising in the management of this type of wound.

Gray reported on the outcome of 1,009 cases of compound fracture of the femur using the Thomas Splint at the Battle of Arras, which was fought during the months of April and May 1917. The Thomas Splint was employed exclusively to immobilise the fracture. Table 4.1 summarises the figures for Gray's cases, comparing his results with outcomes before the Thomas Splint was used routinely.

Following the publication of Gray's book *The Early Treatment of War Wounds* in 1919, based on a series of scientific papers written by Gray and published during the war, Sir Anthony Bowlby attempted to discredit the evidence for the high mortality rate of compound fractures of the femur in the early years of the conflict, declaring it to

---

32 Once in the CCS, glue was used to make sure the traction apparatus didn't slip. It must have been potentially very unpleasant to have it removed later on.

Table 4.1

BEFORE ARRAS; using variety of splints based on Rifle Splint	AT ARRAS using Thomas Splint exclusively
Majority of cases reached CCS in shock due to blood loss and unfit for wound excision	Only 5% of patients reached CCS in shock due to blood loss; majority fit for wound excision
Mortality in CCS 50%; many died before reaching CCS. Total mortality 80%	Mortality 15.6% in CCS
There was a school of thought that all compound fractures of the femur should be treated by amputation, as patients were so moribund- a quick whiff of gas and an amputation gave the only chance of survival	Gray's amputation rate 17.2%. These patients had often lain in a shell hole for many hours and were beyond limb salvage.

Data from Gray, H.M.W., *The Early Treatment of War Wounds*. London: Henry Frowde and Hodder & Stoughton, 1919, pp. 59–60.

have been only sixteen per cent at casualty clearing stations in 1915.[33] Gray issued a robust response in the British Medical Journal, criticising the very inaccurate and misleading figures Bowlby had employed in arriving at his mortality of sixteen per cent.[34] He pointed out that Bowlby's figures had been based on data in admission books at casualty clearing stations. The diagnoses entered in these books were frequently inaccurate, especially during battle periods. At the three casualty clearing stations used by Bowlby in his series, only 141 cases of fractured femur were recorded. There were twenty-three

---

33 Bowlby, A., The Mortality of Cases of Fractured Femur. *British Medical Journal* 1919; 1:p. 112.
34 Gray, H.M.W., The Mortality of Cases of Fractured Femur. *British Medical Journal* 1919; 1: p. 142.

deaths, giving a mortality of sixteen per cent. This was a much smaller number of fractures than would have been expected to have occurred during that period, given the total number of casualties admitted. The accepted incidence of the wound was one case per fifty to sixty admissions. Bowlby should have had an additional 500 cases on which to base his mortality assessment. Gray concluded that Bowlby's figures were extremely flawed, having been based on inaccurate data, and he had probably missed 500 cases which should have been included. Gray had assessed his mortality percentage on a careful study of all cases.

Gray went on to say that it was a pity Bowlby had attempted to diminish appreciation of the excellent progress which had been made in the handling of such cases.

> Had his remarks gone unchallenged, then those who had not given serious consideration to the matter would receive a wrong impression of the appalling seriousness of this injury, especially in the early years of the war.[35]

Once again, Gray had crossed swords with Bowlby. It will become apparent that one of the main criticisms levelled against Gray was that he frequently failed to get on with his contemporaries. This would become a major contributory factor to his ultimate surgical downfall.

Gray's management of penetrating wounds of the knee joint

Gray made a major contribution to improving the prognosis of penetrating wounds of the knee joint.[36, 37] The outcome of these wounds in the early part of the war was very poor indeed and was frequently associated with loss of limb or life. Gray wrote:

---

35 *Ibid.*
36 Gray, H.M.W., Treatment of Gunshot wounds of the knee Joint. *British Medical Journal*; 1915; 2: pp. 41–43.
37 Gray, H.M.W., Gunshot wounds of the knee joint. *British Medical Journal*; 1917; 2: pp. 278–280.

At the record of a healed stiff joint one felt almost inclined to cheer, while the story of movement following an operation sounded like a fairy tale.[38]

Early surgery and the thoroughness of the procedure were vital, as was the ability to close the wound in the joint primarily. The basic principle of surgery for wounds of the knee joint was exactly the same as for other wounds. Complete excision of devitalised tissue and foreign material was of paramount importance and primary closure of the wound was essential to save the joint and retain movement. If infection became established, it usually resulted in disintegration of the joint and breakdown of the patient's general resistance, so that amputation was the only way to save the patient's life.

Soldiers with penetrating wounds of the knee joint were transferred promptly to a casualty clearing station in a Thomas Splint and metallic foreign bodies such as bullets or fragments of shrapnel were localised using x-rays, which helped in the planning of the procedure. For radical limb sparing conservative surgery, great experience was required to excise the wound adequately and yet still be able to close the joint, if not completely, then by stitching the synovial lining[39] of the joint, thus excluding it from the 'outside world' and reducing the risk of infection. Patients whose wounds were associated with major fractures or vessel damage were best treated by immediate amputation. For others, complete wound excision and primary closure usually brought good results.

---

38 Gray, H.M.W., *The Early Treatment of War Wounds*. London: Henry Frowde and Hodder & Stoughton, 1919, p. 254.
39 The synovium is a membrane which lines the inside of a joint. It produces synovial fluid to lubricate the joint. Even if the skin could not be closed completely, if the synovium could be closed across the joint, then all would be well. In later wars plastic surgical procedures became available to provide more reliable soft tissue cover of the joint.

Now, what were fairy tales are commonplace, and great is the satisfaction to those who were out in the dark days of surgery.[40]

Gray's ground breaking work on wound shock

Henry Gray was very aware of the clinical manifestations of shock, since so many patients with compound fractures of the femur reached casualty clearing stations in 1914 and 1915 in a state of circulatory collapse due to blood loss. There was no proper understanding of the clinical condition of shock in the early months of the war and it would be some time before the modern concept of haemorrhagic shock was fully understood.

Modern understanding of shock due to severe blood loss (haemorrhagic shock)

A healthy young man can lose up to thirty per cent of his blood volume without a change in blood pressure and only a modest rise in pulse rate. He can compensate for even larger amounts of blood loss by constricting the blood flow to the skin and other organs, most notably the kidneys. This does two things. By diverting blood away from the skin and kidneys, the supply of vital oxygen-carrying blood to the heart and brain can be maintained, for a while at least. The diversion of blood away from the skin also helps to decrease heat loss and conserve core temperature. In the early months of the war, before measures were taken to keep casualties warm, the core temperature of patients must have fallen. We now know that cardiac output (the amount of blood pumped with every contraction of the heart muscle) falls directly with a decrease in body temperature. The use of motor ambulance wagons which were heated were of great benefit in warming casualties in the journey between the ADS and CCS and improving their clinical condition.[41]

---

40 Gray, H.M.W., *The Early Treatment of War Wounds*. London: Henry Frowde and Hodder & Stoughton, 1919, p. 254.
41 Robertson, E.A., in Scotland, T., and Heys, S., *War Surgery 1914–18*. Solihull: Helion and Co., 2012, pp. 101–104.

When the compensatory mechanisms are inadequate for the blood loss sustained, the ability to preserve the blood pressure is lost and the shock worsens. If the blood pressure falls much below 60mm Hg then the brain is no longer perfused and vital centres of the brain that maintain life stop working. If a patient survives for any length of time with a very low blood pressure, it may be difficult or impossible to reverse.[42]

Severely wounded soldiers needed fluid, blood, warming and early operative intervention. Gray appreciated these requirements in patients with compound fractures of the femur. The Thomas Splint greatly improved the prognosis for this most serious of wounds by effectively immobilising the fracture, limiting blood loss and reducing shock. Surgery performed at CCSs located as close as possible to the front line shortened the transport time from ADSs, thus facilitating early surgery.

To co-ordinate research and clinical observation, the Medical Research Committee[43] (MRC) in 1917 appointed a Special Investigative Committee to look into the problems associated with shock. It consisted of surgeons who were working at casualty clearing stations, supported by physiologists in Britain carrying out research and laboratory doctors at base hospitals. One of those on the Committee was Henry Gray. The full constitution of the Committee was as follows: Professor W.M. Bayliss, FRS; Professor F.A. Bainbridge; Lieut.-Colonel W.B. Cannon, MORC, USA: Dr H.H. Dale, FRS; Colonel T.R. Elliott, FRS, RAMC; Captain John Fraser, RAMC: Colonel H.M.W. Gray, RAMC: Dr P.P. Laidlaw, FRS; Major A.N. Richards; Professor C.S. Sherrington, FRS: Professor E.H. Starling, FRS: Major-General Cuthbert S. Wallace, AMS (T).[44]

As knowledge increased, so did the understanding of shock, as the following quotation from the official Australian Medical History of the war reveals.

---

42 *Ibid.*
43 Medical Research Committee renamed the Medical Research Council on 1 April, 1920.
44 Butler, A.G., *op. cit.*, p. 953.

> Shock as seen in war is usually the result of one or more of the following factors. . . . Shock may be (a) primary or (b) secondary. (a) Primary shock comes on almost immediately after the receipt of the wound. The patient passes into a state of collapse. . . . At this stage the pulse rate and blood pressure may or may not show a great departure from the normal.
>
> (b) Secondary shock manifests itself later . . . Both (a) and (b) are greatly aggravated by loss of blood, sepsis (sic), and mental perturbation. Gray (*Early treatment of War Wounds* 1919, p 81) finds it necessary to distinguish between two conditions, namely, primary shock or the collapse immediately supervening on the infliction of a severe wound and secondary shock, which develops later as the result of such factors as exposure to cold, pain, haemorrhage, movement, anxiety, exhaustion, and all the other harmful influences associated with a long journey to the casualty clearing station.[45]

Gray's influence on shock management became a driving force for Captain Kenneth Walker to establish a 'shock centre' at CCS 3 at Gézaincourt, which was one of the casualty clearing stations of the Third Army for which Gray was responsible. In turn, this inspired Australian medical officer Dr Alan Holmes à Court from the nearby 4th Australian Field Ambulance, to establish a field ambulance resuscitation team to treat the wounded at advanced dressing stations. His team had two medical officers. One was in charge of blood transfusion and capable of performing rapid urgent surgery. The other was experienced in nitrous oxide/oxygen anaesthesia, which was rapidly reversible and did not delay the transfer of wounded soldiers.[46] This second officer was also experienced in resuscitation and blood grouping. There were four non-medical personnel trained in general resuscitation techniques and the team had supplies of all

---

45 Butler, A.G., *op. cit.*, p. 338.
46 Some anaesthetics take a longer time to 'wear off' which would have been very disadvantageous in an ADS where there was an urgent need to ship the wounded out as quickly as possible.

necessary equipment. The following statement comes from the Official Australian Medical History.

> At the front, early in 1918, at No. 3 British CCS at Gézaincourt (Third Army), under the Consulting Surgeon (Colonel Gray), Captain Kenneth Walker,[47] RAMC (T.), had built up a 'Shock Centre,' using whole blood for transfusion, which became a Mecca for front line medical officers, among them a number from the near-by Australian Corps. From these came the idea of field ambulance resuscitation teams.[48]

The Australian Corps, comprising five divisions, expanded the resuscitation team concept over the following months, delivering life saving surgical care at advanced dressing stations.

Gray's other contributions to surgery during the war

Gray published work on the treatment of infected gunshot wounds[49] and gunshot wounds of the head, where once again, the principle of early excision of devitalised tissue was the same and where primary closure of the wound over the brain was essential.[50] He also wrote a paper on gunshot wounds of the spinal cord.[51] He held very strong views on prevention and treatment of gas gangrene which was a direct extension of his pioneering work on wound excision.[52] If all devitalised tissue was radically removed and if there was no dead muscle left in a wound, then the patient would not develop gangrene. By the same token, if the patient had gangrene, then he could only

---

47 Gray paid particular credit to Captain Walker in *The early treatment of war wounds*.
48 Butler, A.G., *op. cit.*, p. 662.
49 Gray, H.M.W., General Treatment of Infected Gunshot Wounds. *British Medical Journal* 1915; 2: pp.41–43.
50 Gray, H.M.W., Gunshot Wounds of the Head. *British Medical Journal* 1916; 1: pp. 261–265.
51 Gray, H.M.W., Early Treatment of Gunshot Injuries of the Spinal Cord. *British Medical Journal* 1917; 2: pp. 44–45.
52 Gray, H.M.W., An essential principle in the treatment of gas gangrene. *British Medical Journal* 1918; 1: p. 369.

be saved by the excision of all dead tissue, although even then he might die from multiple organ failure as a result of the effects of the toxin released by the responsible organisms.

A very rare surgical procedure

Gray removed a bullet from a soldier's heart under local anaesthetic, which illustrates that he, like all others surgeons of his generation, was a surgeon in the most general sense with wide ranging skills.[53] The soldier had been wounded eight days previously with a small wound to the right side of the lower part of his breast bone. A chest x-rays suggested that a bullet was lodged within the muscle wall of the heart, since it moved as the heart was beating. Gray operated under local anaesthetic and made an incision on the front of the chest wall over the breast bone, following the track he thought the bullet would have followed. He held the heart and felt the bullet, which was either within the wall of the right ventricle or lying inside the cavity of the pumping chamber. He took hold of the heart and cut into its muscle to remove the bullet and then stitched the heart muscle back together whilst holding it between his finger and thumb. The operation was completed with the patient feeling no pain. The casualty was well for four hours after the surgery, but then his respiratory rate was observed to be 48 per minute and he died almost five days later. At post-mortem examination the heart was well healed and there was no blood in the pericardial sac.[54] However, there were some clots of blood in the cavity of the right side of the heart and these had become dislodged and travelled to the lungs, blocking the lungs circulation and causing death. This is called a pulmonary embolus.

The personal impact of the war on Gray

Gray's contribution to war surgery was second to none. He pioneered

---

53 Birkbeck, L.H.C., Lorimer, G.N., Gray, H.M.W., Removal of a Bullet from the Right Ventricle of the Heart under Local Anaesthesia. *British Medical Journal* 1915; 2: pp. 561–562.
54 The pericardium is a membrane which completely surrounds the heart.

wound excision, which remains to this day a fundamental principle of war surgery. He developed acute orthopaedic services on the Western Front and saved many lives. His skills and expertise were widely sought after and appreciated, as demonstrated by the high esteem in which he was held by the New Zealand and Australian Medical Services, whose official medical histories both refer to Gray in very positive terms. John Lynn-Thomas from Cardiff, Consulting Surgeon and Deputy Inspector of Military Orthopaedics, Western Command, spoke very highly of Gray, acknowledging his major contribution to the management of septic wounds of the limbs.[55] Gray's diligence and total commitment to his duties earned him the respect of young surgeons working under his instruction and as already stated he was mentioned in dispatches on five occasions.

While focusing on his many achievements, it is easy to lose sight of the fact that working under such arduous conditions for three and a half years must have placed Gray under considerable strain. His hectic work schedule during the time he was in Rouen was interrupted from time to time by brief bouts of ill health, which he mentioned in letters home to his wife Kate in Aberdeen. He was especially prone to back pain, which he attributed to many long hours spent standing and bending over patients on the operating table. He was frequently very tired, since he commonly spent twelve to fourteen hours a day working in the operating theatre and often longer when a particularly heavy load of casualties arrived during a major offensive. Given the sustained level of concentration required for the many taxing surgical procedures he performed on a daily basis, fatigue was inevitable.

In a letter to Eva, in India,[56] dated 24 April 1915, Kate expressed concern over some news from Gray about his health.

---

[55] Thomas, J. Lynn., A simple modification of the Guillotine or Flapless method of Amputation. *British Medical Journal*, 1916; 2: pp. 481–482.

[56] Eva was in India, since her husband, H.T.C. Ivens, the co-author's grandfather, was an officer in the Indian Army, and served in Mesopotamia (modern day Iraq) during the Great War.

Henry is not very well just now but I think he is overdone and tired and is feeling the damp bad weather they have lately had. He wrote not to be alarmed if I had a note saying he was in hospital as he felt he was in for lumbago. I wish he could get home for a bit.

Gray, like many others at the time, also suffered terrible personal loss which affected him deeply. In April 1916, he heard of the death of his brother John, fourteen years his junior. John was killed in action at Kut-el-Amara in Mesopotamia (now known as Iraq) on 11 April 1916, serving with the 36th Sikhs. He was thirty-one years old. He left behind Lucy, his young wife and childhood sweetheart, who was in Darjeeling in India at the time of John's death.

Lucy (nee Henderson), received a telegram[57] stating that her husband was missing. A day later she heard that his body had been found. It was particularly poignant that after several miscarriages during her six-year marriage to John, she was expecting their first child.[58]

News of John's death reached Gray in France via a cable from his elder brother, Aleck, in Aberdeen. Since the death of their parents, John had in many ways been like a son to Aleck and Henry who were much older (eighteen and fourteen years respectively).[59] They took a keen interest in his life and career and like the rest of his family and friends, they were justifiably proud of him. Always an excellent student and accomplished sportsman, John had been an outstanding cadet who earned the Sword of Honour upon graduating from Sandhurst in 1905. He died a fine soldier who had clearly been destined for great things, but in the minds of all who knew him well, it was for his endearing character that he was most mourned. Imbued

---

57 Lucy expressed worry in a telegram to the co-author's grandmother that they wouldn't be able to find the body, and thus not know how he had died.
58 John Willoughby Gray became an actor of some note. The co-author met him in about 1960. He died in 1993.
59 There really were two families within the Gray family unit due to John and Eva being so much younger. This explains the responsibility Gray felt for his younger siblings.

with the Gray family ethos of duty, honesty and selflessness, tempered by a very good sense of humour, John was also endowed with an exceptionally compassionate and affectionate nature. His loss caused Gray profound sadness. Gray wrote a letter of condolence to Eva (Eva Esther Gray Ivens, the co-author's grandmother).

Though Eva was much younger than Gray, he kept in touch with her (often through Kate when he was busy), and there was a great deal of affection between them. He knew only too well what the news of their brother's death must mean for Eva since she and John, who were only one year apart, had been inseparable as children and had remained very close friends to the end. As for Lucy, Gray admitted to being at a loss for words. He could think of nothing he could say that would not fall short of the mark and he asked Eva to tell her so. Lucy had been John and Eva's childhood friend in Aberdeen and he knew her extremely well. Gray had recently heard about Lucy's 'happy prospect' as the family called it and this brought him some consolation, but John's death was quite simply devastating to him. Lucy and Eva remained in touch right up until Lucy's death in 1950.

Gray's letter is reproduced here. There is a reference to Henry and Eva's nephew, Colin Coote, who had caught 'flu in the trenches and who was located by Henry in one of the hospitals in Rouen after much effort, despite Gray's overwhelming workload. The letter also provides some insight into Gray's innermost thoughts. He cursed the war, mentioning the terrible cases he had to see and saying there was worse to come. Towards the end of the letter there is a reference to 'Ivanhoe', who was the co-author's grandfather, Harold Ivens. The nickname comes from his surname Ivens. Gray tentatively asked if Eva still had Ivanhoe with her. Ivanhoe, an officer in the Indian Army, was indeed still with Eva, but was about to embark for Mesopotamia, where like John, he might become a casualty and be killed or wounded.

C/O D.D.M.S.
Rouen
26/iv/16

My Dear Lil Eva,

What a blow to us all is John's death! When I feel it as I do-how much more to poor Lucy and you. I can't bring myself to write to Lucy, but just tell her will you? Damn this war. It gets on my nerves so much, going round as I do, seeing all the worst cases-and the worst is to come!

I have been seedy for the past fortnight. My gee (I was out riding at 6.30 every morning) came down with me and I was knocked out apparently for a bit-and then having to carry on has made me get into a condition that I applied for a fortnight's leave and am going home in 3 days.[60]

You will have heard about Colin – 2 attacks of flu and a devil of a time for especially the past month in the trenches we took over from the French when they moved out between the 1st and the 3rd May to reinforce Verdun, knocked himself up and his heart! Like so many is a little bit dickey but he will be alright in a few weeks. You would hardly have known the boy when I saw him in hospital here – a dreadful strained haunted look in his eyes-but very cheery and distressed to have to come away.

About your dear Baba – I am afraid I can't advise much. You seem to be very sensible about her. If she shows signs of colitis again, I should give her a dose of castor oil with three or four drops of laudanum in it right away and be guided by your own experience after that what to do.[61]

---

60   Aware that he was in need of fresh air and exercise to face each punishing day, Gray had taken to riding his horse at 6.30 am every day before work. The animal had stumbled and fallen throwing Gray, who suffered a brief concussion that left him groggy and bruised, with *a brute of a head*. Three days later he was granted two weeks' leave in Aberdeen.
61   Three year old Barbara was prone to recurrent bouts of colic. Gray had previously provided advice.

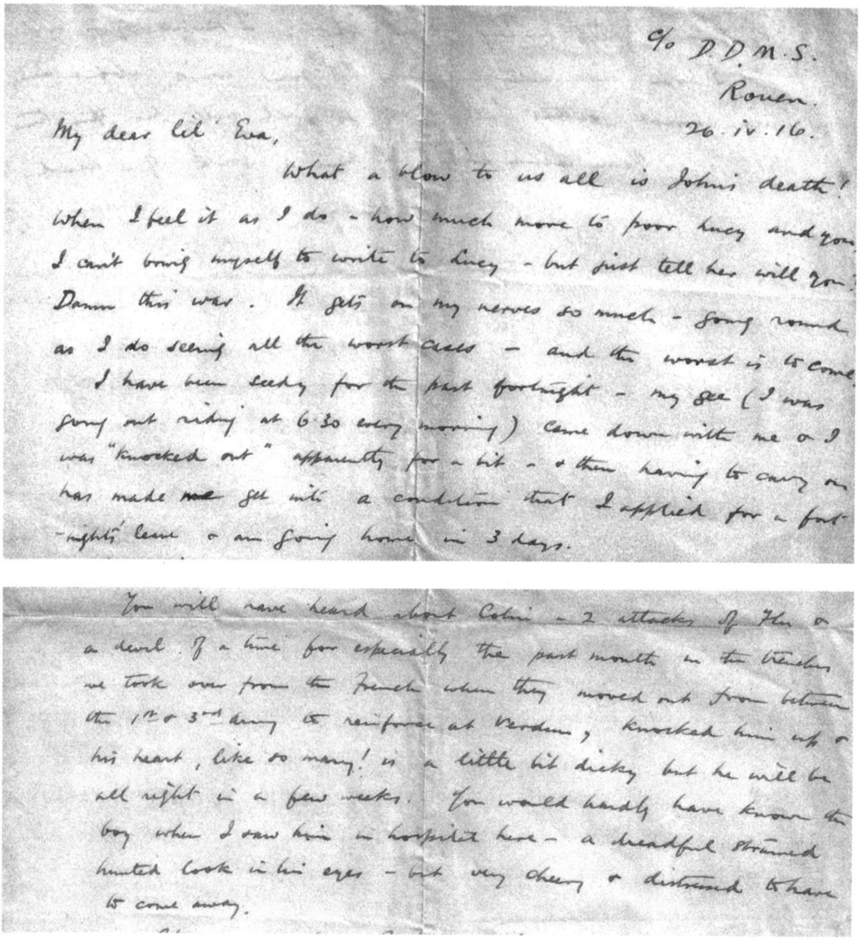

Henry Gray

FIGURE 4.6a and 4.6b
Extracts from Henry Gray's letter to his sister Eva.

I hope you still have Ivanhoe with you. Best love to both of you and keep smiling old girl. I know you will. I hope our interpretations of your wire about Lucy are correct and that all will go well with her this time.

Please excuse more. I have a brute of a head.
Henry.

In this chapter reference has been made to Gray's book, *The Early Treatment of War Wounds*. Colonel Michael Stewart[62] was kind enough to write the foreword for a previous book written by the orthopaedic co-author.[63] During their correspondence, Colonel Stewart made the following statement about Henry Gray, which is a fitting way to summarise his outstanding contribution to war surgery, which is as relevant today as it was one hundred years ago.

> Through three and a half years of concentrated experience of war wounds on a scale hitherto unimaginable, and in collaboration with many brilliant young surgeons, he was able to define the principles of treatment of modern war surgery. One cannot overstate the importance of Sir Henry Gray's book *The Early Treatment of War Wounds*. I do not think there is another text on war surgery that has since bettered it. In terms of the casualty evacuation chain, our Role 3 Military Hospital in Camp Bastion is equivalent to a Casualty Clearing Station.

---

62 Colonel Michael P. M. Stewart, CBE, QHS, MBChB (Abdn) FRCS, FRCS Tr & Orth., L/RAMC, formerly Honorary Surgeon to H.M. The Queen, Consultant Trauma and Orthopaedic Surgeon, and lately Defence Medical Services Consultant Advisor in Trauma and Orthopaedics to the Surgeon General.

63 Scotland, T. and Heys, S., *War Surgery, 1914–18*. Solihull: Helion and Company Limited, 2012.

CHAPTER 5

Gray's career after the Great War

Young surgeons honour Gray with a celebratory dinner in London

On 12 April 1919, Gray was guest of honour at a dinner held at the Criterion Restaurant in London. It was hosted by many of the young surgeons with whom he had worked during the war and as the evening drew to a close, Gray was presented with a large silver bowl as a token of the great admiration they felt for him. Several made speeches and stressed the major contributions Gray had made to surgical progress in the management of war wounds. In reply, Gray said that much of what he had been able to achieve was due to their help. One of those who attended was Captain ETC Milligan, mentioned previously in connection with wound excision. Another present was a Canadian doctor, Lieut. Colonel FA Scrimger, VC, of the Canadian Army Medical Corps,[1] who won his VC during the 2nd Battle of Ypres in 1915. His citation reads:

> On the afternoon of 25th April, 1915 in the neighbourhood of Ypres, when in charge of an advanced dressing station in farm buildings which were being heavily shelled by the enemy, he directed under heavy fire the removal of the wounded and he himself carried a severely wounded officer out of a stable in search of a place of greater safety. When he was unable alone to carry this officer further, he remained with him under fire until help could be obtained. During the very heavy fighting between 22nd and 25th April, Captain Scrimger displayed continuously day and night the greatest devotion to duty amongst the wounded at the front.
>
> *The London Gazette*, 22 June 1915

---

1 Colonel H.M.W. Gray, *British Medical Journal*, 19 April, 1919; p. 503.

The importance of Scrimger's presence at the celebratory dinner will soon become apparent. Gray mentioned the occasion in a letter he wrote to Eva on 14 April, 1919. He also told Eva that he was feeling very tired after all his efforts during the war and was in two minds as to whether to stay in London or go back to Aberdeen after being demobilised.

> Many have been wanting me to start work in London and while I think that I might be able to make good headway, yet there is the feeling that the old bird in the hand is worth as much as ever, that I am not as young as I was, that I have not the same desire to go at full steam, which may return, however, when the tired-out feeling engendered by the war work passes off, that I have not money enough to tide over a possible longish wait for success and at the same time educate the youngsters as I should like.

He went on to say that there were also those who were very keen that he should return to Aberdeen, but it was clear that he had mixed feelings about going back north and financial considerations may have played a part in his final decision.

> People are very keen that I should return to Aberdeen 'for the sake of the (medical) school', although the school does not take much notice of me and the 'call of the north' in various other ways is very strong.

His letter to Eva certainly revealed that he was not particularly enthusiastic at the prospect of going back to his home city and he probably felt very strange when he set foot in Aberdeen Royal Infirmary after an absence of four years. Many things must have changed. Evidence also emerges from the literature that he remained embittered against the surgical establishment in London. In 1921, he delivered an address in Dundee entitled *The application of the professional lessons of the war to civil work*, in which he said that his experience during the war led him to conclude that improvements in medical education were necessary to enable doctors to deal with war

FIGURE 5.1
Henry Gray in later life.

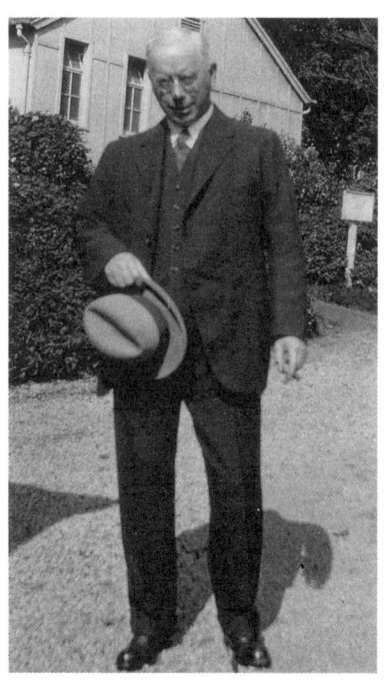

wounds more adequately in future conflicts.[2] With a better education, the average Scottish medical student would have 'greater prowess in the arenas of the world.' He conceded that he himself 'belonged to the ultimate division in the Sassenach classification of those north of the Tweed – the Scotsman, the damned Scotsman and the Aberdonian!'

Then in 1923, Gray was presented with an opportunity for a new challenge. He was approached by a Dr George Armstrong who was soon to retire from the position of Surgeon-in-Chief at the Royal Victoria Hospital in Montreal. Armstrong had come on a mission to the 'Old Country' to find a suitable replacement for himself and Gray was the chosen candidate. Sir Henry Vincent Meredith, President of the Royal Victoria Hospital, was the instigator of Armstrong's overture. Meredith was keen to fill the position of Surgeon-in-Chief quickly. The RVH was short of money and a Surgeon-in-Chief with a busy surgical practice would help to keep the hospital financially solvent.[3] The position usually carried senior status at McGill University. Indeed Armstrong was also Professor of Surgery at McGill. He had served with the Canadian Army Medical Corps in 1916–1917 and knew Gray, but not well.[4]

---

2 Gray, H.M.W., 'An address on the application of the professional lessons of the war to civil work.' *British Medical Journal*, Jan. 22, 1921; pp.109–114.
3 Hanaway, J., Cruess, R., Darragh, J., *McGill Medicine Volume 2, 1885–1936*. Montreal: McGill-Queen's University Press, 2006, pp.112–113.
4 *Ibid.*

Gray's outstanding military surgical career is never mentioned in *McGill Medicine*, which is a two volume history of McGill University, so it would seem as though the medical establishment in Montreal knew very little, if anything, about him.[5] It would also appear that no one in Montreal knew why Gray had been knighted.[6] It has even been suggested that he had been knighted during the war for surgical contributions of a questionable nature.[7]

This is surprising, since Gray was already well established by 1916 as a leading military consulting surgeon. One of those working at the Royal Victoria Hospital after the war was Francis Alexander Scrimger, who returned to work there in 1919 after attending Gray's celebratory dinner in London. Scrimger would spend his remaining career at the RVH and would eventually become Surgeon-in-Chief and Professor of Surgery at McGill University in 1936. He would certainly have had full knowledge of Gray's prowess as a war surgeon and why he had been knighted.

Gray goes to Montreal and meets Sir Arthur Currie

Gray travelled to Montreal, where Dr Armstrong introduced him to Sir Arthur Currie on 27 February 1923. Currie was the Principal and Vice-chancellor of McGill University and had been the exceedingly capable and successful leader of the Canadian Corps during the last eighteen months of the Great War, commanding the Canadians at Passchendaele in 1917 and leading them most successfully at the battle of Amiens in August 1918 and at the Canal du Nord in October 1918.

On 28 February, Currie wrote in his diary that Gray was keen to know what his academic position at McGill University would be.[8]

---

5   *Ibid.*
6   *Ibid.*, p. 115.
7   Entin, M.A., Hanaway, J., Nimeh, T., 'The Principal and the Dean'. Artefacts and Archives/Archives et artefacts de la pratique medicale. *Canadian Bulletin Medical History.* 2003; 20(1): p 161.
8   It is very likely that Armstrong told Gray that the position of Surgeon-in-Chief at RVH carried high University status.

Currie was clearly taken aback by Gray's enquiry and told Gray that he had never been informed about his visit and that until Dr Armstrong resigned, there was no vacancy and nothing could be done. Furthermore, Currie made it very clear that a Selection Board would decide on Armstrong's successor. The Selection Board comprised representatives from the University, from the RVH and from Montreal General Hospital, (MGH). Currie had been placed in a very difficult position and explained to Gray that medical personnel at MGH were of the opinion that McGill medical policy was dictated by the RVH, and that Gray's appearance would confirm their suspicions. Those at MGH would regard the whole affair as a plot.

Currie then met with Sir Henry Vincent Meredith, who apart from being President of the RVH, was also President of the Bank of Montreal. Meredith tried to persuade Currie that the University really ought to jump at the chance of appointing Gray to the Chair of Surgery. Meredith, however, was acting in dictatorial way and was trying to impose Gray on the University without any preliminary discussion. Currie firmly believed that the University could not be dictated to in this way and Gray's impending appointment as Surgeon-in-Chief to the RVH would reflect a definite lack of harmony and co-operation between the University, the Royal Victoria Hospital and Montreal General Hospital.

On 7 March, Currie chaired a meeting of the Medical Advisory Committee. He pointed out that it was the remit of the Committee to recommend who should be offered a University position when a vacancy arose. When a decision had been reached, then the Board of Governors of the University would be informed, as would the Presidents of the RVH and MGH. Currie declared that the RVH had taken it as its right to fill any position on its own staff as it saw fit, without reference to the University, effectively making the University subservient to the RVH. Conversely, when there was an academic vacancy, the University could not appoint anyone it thought suitable unless the RVH was prepared to give a nod of approval and grant the necessary facilities for student teaching and give access to patients.[9] Meredith informed the Advisory Committee that he had given Gray his word that he would be in touch with an offer of the position of Surgeon-in-Chief at the RVH within ten days and he intended to honour it. He was persuaded to have any public announcement withheld for three months to give the University time to make investigations into Gray's suitability for the Chair of Surgery.

Currie obtains references to assess Gray's suitability for the Chair of Surgery

Currie began to gather information about Gray. He wrote to the Principals and Vice-chancellors of the Universities in Scotland, asking about Gray's suitability for an academic position. The Principals in turn asked appropriate individuals who knew Gray to provide references. The names of the referees have been withheld by McGill Archives for reasons of confidentiality but here is a general summary of their collective assessments.

The referees had not found it an easy matter. There were two distinct components to Gray's professional profile. On the one hand, he was an able and strong man. There was no doubt about his professional qualities. He was a surgeon of considerable originality and was full of ideas. He was of upright character and displayed frankness and courage. He held and never disguised strong opinions. One referee stated that he was not the type of individual to quarrel with others for holding different views, but others disagreed with this statement. He had a reputation for being a brilliant and original surgeon and was largely responsible for phenomenal developments in joint surgery, thoracic surgery and the management of head injuries during the war. No one had done such good work for the Third Army and there was close co-operation between the army commander and Gray. One referee stated that he was the best consulting surgeon

---

9 The unilateral action of Meredith in seeking out and appointing Gray to the position of Surgeon-in-Chief at RVH without reference to the University became a major battleground between Currie and Meredith.

in the British Army. He was frank and open in controversy. He was a keen, fertile thinker, but was never too quick to change from old established principles to new methods. He never spared himself and worked from early in the morning to late at night and was an extremely good operator. He was a charming and loyal man, who given a free hand would organise a notable unit. He had an excellent following among the <u>young surgeons</u> (underlined by the referee) with whom he worked.

On the other hand, Gray was described by one referee as a difficult and complex personality. He was a poor speaker. Another said that Gray was a very old friend and an admirable surgeon but shared acrimonious and difficult relations with some of the authorities. He was intolerant of opposition and suffered from a want of tact; he was a fighter. Henry Gray did the greatest war work at the front, achieving greater practical results than any other surgeon, but his zeal created many enemies among senior colleagues. Gray was 'not at his best on a platform' but the referee making this statement had no direct knowledge of his ability to teach. If taken the right way, Gray might be a success – but how he would be under opposition (in Canada) was unknown.

On 19 March, Currie recorded in his diary that a London Professor of Surgery (name has been withheld) called, who stated that they wouldn't raise any flags for Gray in London. His support in the army had come from younger men. Gray found it difficult to get on with colleagues; he was too arbitrary; too impulsive; too dictatorial; London surgery would regard Archibald superior to Gray.[10]

On 4 April, Currie wrote to the Principal and Vice-Chancellor of

---

10 Born in Montreal, Edward William Archibald was a research-oriented surgeon who trained with Sir Victor Horsley, the British neurosurgeon at Queen's Square, London. He subsequently became Professor of Surgery at McGill in 1923, closing the door on Gray. He would be appointed Chief of Surgery at RVH, but not till 1928.

Liverpool University, Sir George Adami, who was a close friend.[11] Currie told Adami that the information he was getting about Gray was conflicting. On the one hand, there was general agreement that he was a very good surgeon. On the other hand, he was a poor speaker and found it difficult to get on with his senior colleagues. Some had unhesitatingly supported Gray, while other opinions were not at all favourable. Some said Gray was a good administrator, while others said he was not. He certainly had the faculty to stimulate juniors, but all were agreed that Gray was unlikely to get on with his contemporaries. He was a man of very positive views who bitterly resented any opposition.

Currie confided in Adami that he had been accused by Montreal General Hospital of being in league with Meredith in appointing Gray. He went on to say that there was no support from other members of staff at the RVH for Meredith and Armstrong's unilateral action. Indeed, other members of staff at the RVH were bitterly disappointed by the way Armstrong and Meredith had behaved in approaching Gray. Surgeons at MGH were up in arms, while McGill men resented the fact that no McGill surgeon was apparently good enough to be considered for the position of Surgeon-in-Chief. There was only one thing that would make Gray acceptable-and that would be if he was outstandingly qualified for the Professorship of Surgery.

---

11 Sir George Adami (1862–1926) was educated at Owen College, Manchester, and at Christ's College, Cambridge, where he obtained a first class honours in natural science. He subsequently studied in Breslau and Paris He was Darwin prizeman in 1885, MRCS, and was appointed demonstrator of pathology in Cambridge University in 1887. In 1888, he accidentally exposed himself to rabies, and published an account of his treatment at the Pasteur Institute's vaccination clinic. Elected fellow of Jesus College, Cambridge, in 1891, he soon afterwards became head of the pathology department of the Royal Victoria Hospital in Montreal. From 1892, he was Professor of Pathology in McGill University. During the Great War, he inspected Canadian hospitals in France. From 1919, he was Vice-Chancellor of University of Liverpool.

On 9 April, Meredith wrote to Currie informing him that he had cabled Gray, formally offering him the position of Surgeon-in-Chief at RVH and Gray had accepted. Meredith thought that Gray would be ideal for the position of Professor of Surgery at McGill University. He wanted to make a public announcement of Gray's appointment and once again he tried to pressurise Currie to appoint Gray to the Chair of Surgery so that a joint announcement could be made but Currie was having none of it. He felt that he simply must write to Gray to make the University's position absolutely clear, which he did on 11 April. In his correspondence, he said he had received a letter from Sir Henry Vincent Meredith stating that Gray had been offered the position of Surgeon-in-Chief at the RVH and that Gray had accepted. He wanted to make it absolutely clear that being appointed to this position in no way implied that the post automatically went with the headship of the University, nor for that matter with any position on the teaching staff. At the same time, Currie wrote to Meredith, stating that he was not convinced by Gray's credentials for the Chair of Surgery. He had sought opinions from Principals and Vice-chancellors of leading Scottish and English Universities and while Gray was a good operator, none had said he was a good teacher and he had no experience of systematic lecturing. He had no standing as a medical educationalist and there were none who felt his contributions to the surgical literature would outlive his generation or be of permanent value. Gray was a difficult, complex, person and was not the kind of man to work smoothly with colleagues. He was tactless to the extreme and intolerant of opinions of others which differed from his own.

Gray replies to Currie
On 24 April, Gray replied to Currie. He knew that his acceptance of the position of Surgeon-in-Chief at the Royal Victoria Hospital did not imply headship of the McGill University Surgical Department. He went on to say, however, that anyone holding the position of Surgeon-in-Chief would be very involved with student teaching, since

the most important aspect of teaching was ward work.[12] Gray went on to assure Currie that there was no cause for misunderstanding, and that he would do his very best for the University, even indirectly, and that in the long term the University and RVH would feel no cause for regret for appointing him.[13]

The Rockefeller Foundation vetoes Gray for the Professorship of Surgery

On 14 May, Currie recorded that he had been in conversation with a Dr Pierce of the Rockefeller Foundation, who had expressed strong disapproval of the manner of Gray's appointment, stating that as long as the Medical School permitted itself to be dictated to by a hospital it could expect no support from the Rockefeller Foundation. Currie and Dr Charles Martin, the Dean of the Faculty of Medicine at McGill, were involved in delicate negotiations with the Rockefeller Foundation for financial support for a full time Professorship of Medicine and the establishment of a University Clinic at the RVH. When the Rockefeller executives heard that Meredith had ignored McGill's policy and appointed a Surgeon-in-Chief unilaterally, negotiations were put on hold until the University asserted its policies.[14]

Further deterioration in Currie's relationship with Meredith

On 5 June, Currie wrote in his diary that Dr. Martin had just returned from a visit to the Rockefeller Foundation's executives in New York. It transpired that Meredith had already visited them and had told them that Currie, as Principal of the University, had known from the very beginning about the negotiations with Gray. Currie

---

12 This implied that he, Gray, as Surgeon-in-Chief would have control over student access to patients.
13 Gray's response is guarded; perhaps he senses trouble ahead.
14 Hanaway, J., Cruess, R., Darragh, J., *McGill Medicine, Volume 2, op.cit.*, p. 115.

could not understand why Meredith had made this statement, since it was simply not true.[15]

On 17 June, Armstrong visited Currie to say that Meredith was angered by the decision of the University not to give Gray a full professorship. Armstrong urged that this should be done for the sake of harmony and for the sake of future relations between the University and the RVH. Currie replied that there was an important principle at stake. Who controlled University appointments-the hospitals or the University? Currie reminded Armstrong of the Selection Board policy, saying that Archibald would probably be made head of the Surgical Department and Gray would be offered a position on the teaching staff, but not a full professorship. If Gray accepted this, then it would be interpreted as an act of good will and would pave the way to better relationships. Whether Gray would achieve full professorship would depend on his attitude after his arrival.[16]

---

15 This is a reflection of the very poor relationship between Currie and Meredith. There is nothing in the McGill documents to suggest that Currie knew about Gray; quite the opposite in fact. It would seem that Meredith was out to make mischief between the Rockefeller Foundation and the Principal.

16 This was a move on the part of the University to negate Meredith's aspirations to have Gray made Professor of Surgery. By getting Archibald installed as Professor of Surgery, Meredith would be thwarted. The move would also keep the Rockefeller Foundation happy. Indeed, on 20 June, Currie wrote that he had had a meeting in New York with Dr Pierce of the Rockefeller Foundation. The foundation was very positive that there should be a re-assertion of adherence to the principle behind the Selection Board. Gray should not be offered any appointment with the University until he came and the University had the chance to assess what his attitude would be. They thought he ought to be satisfied with a clinical professorship and that indeed any position on the teaching staff of the University ought to satisfy him.

Sir Edward Beatty visits Britain and tries to persuade Gray to accept a clinical professorship

Sir Edward Beatty was Chancellor of McGill University and was also President of the Canadian Pacific Railway. He was in Britain on a visit when Currie sent him a cable on 23 June, requesting him to make contact with Gray and to suggest that it would be greatly to Gray`s advantage if he were to confirm that a full professorship was not expected. A couple of days later, he sent another cable, saying that there would be no hope of progress as long as the RVH insisted on a full professorship for Gray. If Gray were to put in writing that he did not want a full professorship and would accept an annually renewable clinical professorship (which would be junior to the Professor of Surgery), then that would be helpful; it would break the deadlock.[17]

On 28 June, Beatty replied to Currie, saying that he had been unable to meet with Gray. He would have much preferred speaking to him in person, but apparently it had been impossible for Gray to make an appointment. Beatty wrote to Currie again on 9 July, saying he had tried unsuccessfully to get Gray to meet him in Liverpool. As things stood, Gray would not commit himself beyond the very non-specific letter he had written to the Principal on 24 April. Beatty pointed out that Gray was not at all familiar with the situation in Montreal and thought that Currie would have to explain the political background to Gray to make sure he understood exactly what was going on, so that he could prepare himself and take such steps as necessary to reduce the likelihood of friction after his arrival in Montreal.[18]

---

17 Such a move would go a long way to resolving the problem Currie was having with the Rockefeller Foundation.
18 All this political maneuvering was going on while Gray was still in Aberdeen. He had not yet taken up his appointment.

Meeting of Electoral Board to pick successor to Dr Armstrong

On 19 July a meeting of the Electoral Board was held to choose a successor to Dr Armstrong as Head of Surgery. Meredith declined to attend, giving the reason that there was no mention on the agenda of his letter of 12 May.[19] Archibald was duly appointed to the Chair of Surgery. His name was put forward by Dr Armstrong, whose proposal was duly seconded and the appointment approved.[20]

Gray arrives in Montreal to take up his position of Surgeon-in-Chief at RVH

A further meeting of the Electoral Board was planned to take place on 6 August, to discuss the possible offer of a teaching position to Gray. Once again, Meredith declined to attend, giving the same reason as before. Currie postponed this meeting of the Electoral Board because Gray had now arrived in Montreal.

On 12 September, Martin wrote to Gray, offering him an associate professorship of surgery, explaining that a full professorship was simply not possible, since such an appointment would endanger the future of McGill Medical School. If Gray accepted an associate professorship, then it would be seen as a conciliatory move on his part and would go a long way towards promoting harmony. Martin also said that should Gray refuse the offer, then it would be greatly disadvantageous, so he hoped Gray would cooperate to help everyone concerned out of a very serious predicament.

Gray replied to Martin a couple of days later. He had decided not to accept the University position which had been offered. He was

---

19 On 12 May, Meredith wrote to Currie and suggested the University should appoint Archibald to be Chairman of the Surgical Department of McGill and offer Gray a Professorship of Surgery. Currie replied on 19 July, saying that Meredith's letter contained suggestions that could only be dealt with by Electoral Board and by Board of Governors of University.

20 It is interesting to note that Armstrong proposed Archibald. It may seem absurd to the present day observer that Armstrong had so much to do with the appointment of his successor.

willing to give clinical instruction to the best of his ability, should it be desired, without academic title. He also gave assurance that he would further McGill's interests from an independent position. Gray ended by asking Martin if he would send him the teaching programme for the following year for his approval.

Currie wrote to Gray on 22 September, clearly very upset by his refusal to accept an associate professorship, declaring that he was extremely disappointed by his attitude. Currie asked Gray to reconsider his position otherwise his apparent willingness to co-operate with the University would be mere words and nothing more.[21] Gray wrote to Currie on 23 September, referring him to his letter of the 14th. He had still not received the teaching programme and as Surgeon-in-Chief he reserved the right to see it and approve it, since it had to fit in with the large amount of work to be dealt with in the RVH.[22]

On 24 September, Martin wrote to Gray, saying it was very regrettable that Gray had not accepted an associate professorship. He went on to say that University relied on Gray granting every facility to the University to further the teaching of students in the wards, theatres and laboratories.[23]

1924: marked worsening of relations

There is a gap of one year between the correspondence on 24 September 1923 and the next entry in Currie's diary on 26 September 1924. Clearly relations had not improved. Indeed, there was evidence of a marked deterioration. Gray went to see Currie on that day and

---

21 Currie had realised that as Surgeon-in-Chief, Gray would grant facilities for teaching on conditions laid down by Gray alone, and that Gray could teach from a position independent of the University and therefore out with its control. He would in no way be under the directorship of the Professor of Surgery.
22 Gray was fighting back against the McGill establishment.
23 Martin was seeking assurance from Gray that he would co-operate with student teaching and grant access to the surgical wards and operating theatres in RVH.

informed him that the Medical Faculty was ignoring him and that student teaching programmes were being arranged without his input. Currie told Gray that it was entirely up to the Professor of Surgery to draw up the teaching programme together with the Dean and the surgical staff, after which it should be submitted in writing to the Surgeon-in-Chief (Gray) for his approval. Gray wanted an acknowledgement on the part of the University that the use of RVH facilities for student teaching should be approved by the Surgeon-in-Chief. He also told Currie that certain members of the hospital staff were slandering him, and he proposed to take further formal action.[24]

Charge of Professional misconduct brought by Gray against Dr Martin

Gray was asked to see a patient in the Royal Victoria Hospital by the patient's family.[25] The attending physician did not trust Gray, and asked Dr Martin to give a second opinion. Martin contradicted Gray and this clearly humiliated him. Gray called for an investigation of Martin by the Canadian Medical Association.

On 27 November 1924, Martin wrote to Meredith. Two months had passed since Gray had made a verbal charge of professional misconduct against him in the presence of a witness. Gray had subsequently submitted the charge in writing to the Board of Governors. This written document had been withdrawn as far as he understood and had been left for Chancellor Beatty's consideration. Despite the passing of a couple of months, Martin had heard nothing from Gray about the incident.

Martin stated that the charges should be confirmed, in which case he would respond accordingly, or they should be withdrawn with an apology, otherwise he would have to bring the matter before the

---

24 There is nothing documented to explain what these slanderous actions were, or who perpetrated them.
25 Hanaway, J., Cruess, R., Darragh, J., *McGill Medicine, Volume 2, op.cit.,* pp.116–117.

Medical Faculty and before the Medical Board of the RVH. The Governors of the hospital should inform Gray of his obvious duty to avert a serious crisis and at least restore superficial harmony.

Meanwhile, the question of student timetables had raised its head again as the new term was about to get underway. Gray had sought clarification of his position, maintaining that no discussions for the forthcoming academic year had taken place with him. On 21 October 1924, Archibald wrote to Gray. He summarised the position by saying that Gray had declined any University teaching position below the level of professor. As he understood matters, Gray could not accept a University position which was junior to his junior in RVH (Archibald). Gray's position would remain as a voluntary teacher in an extra-mural position. As far as Archibald was concerned, given that Gray's attitude had not changed, he saw no reason to alter existing arrangements.

On 24 October, Currie wrote to Gray and was clearly exasperated. Archibald had shown him the correspondence he had exchanged with Gray. Appropriate discussions most certainly had taken place. The matter had been discussed in Currie's office on 22 September and again at his house on 26 September. Currie did not know what more could be done, other than put in writing that the University recognised Gray's position as Surgeon-in-Chief at RVH and that it acknowledged what he had done in the 1923–24 session, and what he was going to contribute in the 1924–25 session, and that there was no academic rank.

That evening, Gray sent Currie a hand written letter from his home in which he thanked Currie for his letter of 24 October, confirming that all he wanted was written confirmation of his role. He agreed with everything Currie had said and was happy to continue on the same basis. He wanted everything dealt with before the start of the term and not after it had begun. He assured Currie of his on-going support for McGill and apologised for being indirectly responsible for causing Currie unnecessary trouble.

Descent into an impossible situation

The documents then go on to 30 April 1925. Gray was experiencing major difficulties from the staff at the RVH and was now working from the Medical Arts building of the University. Any opposition the University had ever had to Gray was by now far outweighed by feelings entertained by the Royal Victoria Hospital authorities against him. Gray must at some point have been offered a sum of money if he retired quietly without making a fuss, because Currie alluded to this in a letter, in which he said that Gray had shown no inclination to accept the amount suggested as quid pro quo should he be asked to retire.[26] Currie stated that he was afraid the hospital was not out of the woods with regards to the matter and he referred to Gray as a joker.

The end of the road for Gray

On 22 September 1925, Currie wrote a memo. He had had enough. Following a meeting that morning, he had met with Meredith to talk very frankly with him. Since Gray's appointment as Surgeon-in-Chief to the RVH, a very bad atmosphere had been created and Currie wanted to put a stop to it, both for his own sake and for the sake of the University. Matters had not improved over two years and Currie could see nothing but more trouble ahead. The longer Gray taught without rank and without pay, the greater would be the obligation under which he was placing McGill University. Currie thought the only thing to do would be to free the University from Gray. He wrote to him and asked him to meet with Archibald and himself on 24 September. Following this meeting, Currie wrote to Gray, summarising the views to which he, Currie, had given expression at the meeting.

Currie felt that the existing arrangement for Gray to teach without pay and position was unsound. Currie had acted out of a desire to

---

26 There is no further documentation of this offer of financial settlement if he was to retire.

ease a difficult situation but it hadn't worked and he felt that the arrangement should be terminated. He felt that a very bad atmosphere had been created and wanted rid of it. Members of hospital staff were also members of the University and opinions and loyalties were split, which he felt was a very bad state of affairs. The esprit de corps of the University was at stake. Currie reminded Gray of his army experience. Gray should know the value of esprit de corps.[27]

Currie duly informed Meredith on the same day that the University had terminated its association with Gray, sending Meredith a copy of the letter he had written to Gray. He also sent a copy to Sir Charles Gordon, President of the RVH. Gordon replied, saying the RVH would go along with Currie's decision to remove Gray from the teaching, but this should not be seen as a precedent to affect actions of the RVH in the future.

On 25 September, HE Webster, Secretary RVH, wrote to Gray. The Executive of the Royal Victoria Hospital had reluctantly decided to ask for his resignation as Surgeon-in-Chief. When he resigned, the executive would be prepared to offer him an appointment as a consultant surgeon at the RVH. On 29 September, Gray replied to Webster, saying he preferred to sever connections completely, asking for the return of surgical instruments which belonged to him.

Gray's response to Currie on 28 September: 'The Paranoid rambling letter'[28]

On 28 September, Gray wrote a letter to Currie; declaring that vindication of his position was required, and that publication (of

---

27 This is the first ever reference or acknowledgement made by Currie that Gray had been in the Army.
28 In Hanaway, J., Cruess, R., Darragh, J., *McGill Medicine, Volume 2*, p. 117, the authors refer to a long rambling paranoid letter Gray wrote to the CMAJ, saying that his programmes were being interfered with and that there was a plot against him.

correspondence) was necessary; he thought that Archibald's appointment was a deliberate attempt to undermine him. He re-stated his belief in the benefits of teaching without academic position. He referred to a systematic campaign against him which had formed the subject of common talk in Montreal and was being commented on in the English speaking world. Before completing and posting his letter, the communication from the Board of Governors of RVH arrived, asking for his resignation. Consequently, he sent copies of his letter to the Editor of the Canadian Medical Association Journal. There is a hand written note at the bottom of Gray's letter saying the Editorial Board would not publish it, believing it to be quite unnecessary, and would lead to further unpleasant correspondence.[29]

Gray's further correspondence with the medical press
On 3 October, 1925, the following paragraph was published in the British Medical Journal.

> Telegrams despatched from Montreal on September 29th announce that Sir Henry Gray has found it necessary to resign his position as Surgeon-in-Chief of the RVH in Montreal and also as a clinical lecturer in surgery in McGill University to which he was appointed about two years ago. From the brief abstract telegraphed to the Daily Mail of the correspondence which has taken place between him and General Sir Arthur Currie, Principal of McGill University, it appears that Sir Henry Gray considers that from an early stage, he has not had fair play from his hospital colleagues. When in 1923 he accepted the appointments in Montreal he was surgeon to the Aberdeen Royal Infirmary, where he had resumed duty after acting for several years with the British Army in France, in which capacity he earned a reputation as a surgeon of great independence of judgement and brilliant executive ability. His surgical colleagues in this country will learn with deep regret of his resignation from the offices he held in Montreal.[30]

---

29 *Ibid.*, p. 117.
30 Sir Henry Gray, *British Medical Journal*, 3 October, 1925; p. 621.

This release is documented in the McGill archives, with a hand written note on it to say it was not to appear in their journal (*Canadian Medical Association Journal*).[31]

On 24 October, 1925, the *British Medical Journal* published the following three letters.[32]

First letter:

From Gray to the Editor,

The Canadian Medical Association Journal:

Sir, I feel that the virtual dismissal of one of the chief members of staff of such a well known institute as the RVH, Montreal, must be of interest to the medical profession. I send you the enclosed copy of correspondence for publication in the BMJ. I am not aware of having committed any professional or social action which would merit such dismissal. I am etc., Henry M W Gray

Montreal Oct 9th

Second letter:

From HE Webster, Secretary of RVH on September 25, 1925 to Gray:

Sir Henry Gray, KBE,
Surgeon-in-Chief,
Royal Victoria Hospital, Montreal

Dear Sir Henry,
Sir Arthur Currie has sent the hospital a copy of his correspondence of his letter to you of 24th instant. In view of that letter, and under the circumstances, the executive of the hospital has reluctantly decided to ask you to be good enough to hand in your resignation as Surgeon-in-Chief. When you do so, the executive is prepared to appoint you consulting surgeon to the hospital.

---

31 This was clearly causing considerable consternation. Steps were being taken by McGill to limit any damage caused by Gray's resignation.

32 Sir Henry Gray, *British Medical Journal*, 24 October, 1925; p. 770.

Third letter:

> From Gray to HE Webster, Secretary Board of Governors, RVH, September 29, 1925:
>
> H E Webster Esq.,
> Secretary Board of Governors,
> Royal Victoria Hospital, Montreal
>
> Dear Sir,
> In reply to your letter dated 25th instant, I formally accede to the request of the 'executive of the hospital.' In view of all the circumstances of my connection with the RVH, I prefer to sever my connection with it completely now. I am sorry to trouble you further, but should like to have the instruments etc which I provided for use in the hospital returned or replaced.

While all three letters were published in the British Medical Journal, the Canadian Medical Association Journal only published the second and third. When it did so in November 1925 it also published the following disclaimer:[33]

> In reference to the resignation of Sir Henry Gray, the British Medical Journal of 3 October refers to him as a lecturer of clinical surgery in McGill University. We are informed that McGill University had no part in inviting Sir Henry to come to Montreal, and that at no time did he occupy any position whatever on its staff. Such instruction as he gave was without academic position. We are also informed that the Medical Board of the RVH had no part either in Sir Henry's appointment or in his resignation.[34]

---

[33] Correspondence; Resignation of Sir Henry Gray; *Canadian Medical Association Journal*, November 1925; 15(11): p. 1163.

[34] It is certainly true that McGill University had no part in inviting Gray to come to Montreal. It is also true that he never at any time occupied a position on its staff. It would seem, however, that board members of the RVH were maintaining that they had no part in appointing Gray to the position of Surgeon-in-Chief to RVH. Unable to control the actions of Sir Henry Vincent Meredith, they were attempting to wash their hands of the entire affair.

Correspondence between Currie and Dr George Gibson in Edinburgh[35]

On 28 September 1925, Currie wrote to his good friend Dr George Gibson in Edinburgh. He had recently arrived back in Montreal after a trip they had undertaken together to the Great War battlefields of France and Flanders. After talking about their recent trip Currie went on to ask if Gibson could verify the rumour that there was a trace of insanity in the family of a prominent Montreal surgeon. There had been interesting developments.

On 13 October, Gibson replied, stating that he knew nothing about any history of lunacy in Gray's family; he was meeting a man the following day who might be able to give him more information. He went on to say that the Gray debacle was not of much importance in Britain and Gibson had put one or two people straight about the facts, spreading the news that Gray had had no definite agreement or promise regarding a professorship when he went to Montreal. Gibson had also spoken to a relation of Gray's by marriage and there was no trace of insanity in the family. On 27 October, Gibson wrote again to Currie, stating that he had not heard another word about Gray. He reported that Gray had not even attained the dignity of being a nine-day wonder. He was more like a nine minute one.[36]

Further media attention in the wake of Gray's removal: correspondence between Henry Birks and Currie[37]

On 30 September, Henry Birks, who was a friend with strong McGill connections, and who was visiting Britain, wrote to Currie. Birks

---

35 Dr Gibson lived in Edinburgh and clearly knew Currie well; he went on a trip to the battlefields with Currie; Gibson was tasked with writing an account of their trip and giving it to Blackader, the Editor of the *Canadian Medical Association Journal*. Gibson wrote a regular letter to the CMAJ telling them about medical news from the 'Old Country'.

36 Gibson is reassuring Currie that any fallout from Gray's removal had not had any significant effect in the 'Old Country'.

37 Henry Birks (1840–1928) was a Canadian businessman and founder of

suggested there should be a pre-emptive strike with a carefully worded statement to head off possible media accusations that McGill had engaged in an anti-British policy with the removal of Gray. Such a story would have been good ammunition for many of the newspapers. Birks maintained that if Gray returned to Britain, he would be sure to excuse himself and blame McGill University for everything that had happened. Currie was away in British Columbia at the time and did not reply till 7 November (see below). On 1 October, Birks cabled Currie, suggesting he should make a statement to the Canadian Medical Association Journal to forestall unfair comment and to prevent anti-British accusations being made against McGill.

On 7 November, Currie finally replied to Birks. He had not made any statement to the press and gave his reasons. In the first place, to have done so would have convicted Meredith. The University had won its battle. Meredith had been defeated. The battle had been for a principle, namely the right to say who should constitute University staff and it was over. In the second place, Currie was of the opinion that Gray possessed a cunning cleverness to turn everything around to his advantage and any further correspondence would quite simply prolong the controversy. Currie stressed that the University had had no part in inviting Gray to come to Montreal. They had looked at his qualifications and found a better man in Archibald. Despite being clearly warned, Gray had persisted in coming to Montreal and had endeavoured to force himself onto McGill as its Professor of Surgery.[38]

Henry Birks and Sons, a chain of high-end Canadian jewellery stores. The William and Henry Birks Building at Montreal's McGill University, a Collegiate Gothic structure on University Street, is named in honour of Birks and one of his sons.

38 The Battle of who made University appointments had been fought and won by Currie. In the interests of restoration of order, Currie did not take matters further with Meredith, who was the real villain. Gray's reputation and career were sacrificed. There is no evidence that he tried to force himself upon McGill as their Professor of Surgery. It was Meredith who had tried to force Currie's hand to appoint Gray to the Chair of Surgery.

Correspondence between Dr Casey Wood and Currie, which reveals the feeling of Canadians towards the 'Old Country'[39]

On 7 November, a friend by the name of Dr Casey Wood wrote to Currie. He had met Gray several times in Montreal and shared news of common Aberdeen friends. Wood said he had formed a strong liking for Gray. However, he felt Currie had acted in the best interests of the University. The Canadian part of his makeup really looked forward to the day when Canada would be completely free and independent of Britain. Professorial positions should be filled by individuals who had made Canada their home and not by people passing through. Wood said he might be wrong, but he sensed that the attitude of many McGill alumni was because of a patriotic force and not because of any feeling of personal hostility towards Gray.

On 14 December, Currie replied to Wood, who was in Ceylon. He thanked him for his comments about Gray and said that the English press had behaved unwisely, because it assumed wrongly that bad relations with Gray were because he was from the 'Old Country'. He had not responded to the press because in doing so, he would have had to convict Meredith. He had won his battle, and he refused to enter the field of recrimination. Currie stressed that it was because of the way Gray was brought to Canada and the way he was forced upon the University against its will that aroused feeling against him, and not because he came from the 'Old Country'.

---

39 Dr Casey Wood (1856–1942) was an ophthalmologist, ornithologist and bibliophile. He was born in Wellington, Ontario and obtained his MD from University of Bishop's College (Quebec) in 1877 and McGill in 1906 after the merger of the two medical faculties. In 1911, he presented a large collection of rare books on the subject of diseases of the eye to McGill Medical Library. In 1919, he established The Emma Shearer Wood Library of Ornithology at McGill. After his retirement in 1917, he travelled widely, including to Ceylon. He wrote from Ceylon where he was engaged in archaeological pursuits collecting ancient Ceylonese coinage which he proposed to donate to the Redpath Museum, opened at McGill in 1882, Redpath being the benefactor.

On 23 March 1926, Currie wrote to Professor Williams, who was Professor of History at the University of Edinburgh.[40] Williams had written a supportive letter, published in the Scotsman, combating the view that Old Countrymen were not welcome at McGill.[41]

Present day perception of Gray at McGill University – The Sir Henry Gray Affair

In McGill Medicine, Volume 2, published in 2006, the authors make the point that Meredith ignored the protocol for appointments to McGill teaching hospitals and invited Gray to visit Montreal, but did not acquaint him with the underlying dynamics of the situation.[42] Meredith promised Gray the position of Surgeon-in Chief and persuaded the RVH board to ratify the appointment.[43] He thought he could persuade Currie to make Gray Professor of Surgery, but Meredith was wrong and he greatly overestimated his position and influence. Currie was having none of it, and did not back down. The matter was further complicated when the Rockefeller Foundation executives heard that Meredith had unilaterally ignored McGill appointment policies. Funding matters were put on hold till McGill asserted itself.[44] The authors describe three steps which were taken to deal with Gray, all of which were designed to humiliate him.

The University's first move was to appoint Archibald Professor of Surgery, closing the door on Gray.

McGill's second move was to remove Gray from the student

---

40 Williams became Kingsford Professor of History at McGill University in 1921, and then Professor of history at Edinburgh University from 1925 to 1937 when he retired. In 1935 he was elected a Fellow of the British Academy.
41 A defensive strategy combating anti-British accusation continued for some time after Gray's removal.
42 Hanaway, J., Cruess, R., Darragh, J., *McGill Medicine, Volume 2, op. cit.*, pp. 112–117.
43 It would seem that he bullied them into submission, which does not say much for their professional integrity.
44 The position was quite clear. Gray would have to be removed.

surgical lecture rotation because he was a poor, disorganised teacher. 'This move was calculated to humiliate him (Gray) and did just that'.

'The final challenge to the beleaguered Gray', to use the authors' own words, and described by them as an insensitive man who did not care for McGill tradition, came when Martin contradicted Gray's clinical opinion. 'Gray, again humiliated, called for an investigation of Martin by the CMA'.

Aftermath

The authors of McGill Medicine go on to say that Gray had completely disrupted the RVH department of surgery by attempting to reorganise hospital systems, failing to promote research and refusing to wear surgical gloves. It was standard practice in the Montreal hospitals by then to wear gloves while performing surgical procedures.[45]

Morale in the RVH Department of Surgery was very low after the Gray debacle. The whole wretched affair strengthened McGill's resolve to tighten its policies on appointments. Sir Henry Vincent Meredith's control of hospital affairs declined, but he blocked Archibald's appointment as Surgeon-in-Chief. He never confronted Martin or Currie again. He began to withdraw from his duties as President of the RVH and no longer had absolute control of all matters relating to the hospital. He declined mentally and resigned in 1928.[46]

---

45 Reference has been made previously about Gray's attitude to wearing gloves while operating.
46 Hanaway, J., Cruess, R., Darragh, J., *McGill Medicine, Volume 2, op.cit.*, p. 119.

CHAPTER 6

An appraisal of Gray's surgical career

Factual accounts of the three phases of Gray's 'surgical life' have now been provided, based on existing evidence from the medical literature, as well as in the latter phase from the diaries and correspondence of Sir Arthur Currie from the Archives of McGill University. The aim now is to provide an overall appraisal of Gray's surgical career, exploring the strengths which made him such an outstanding surgeon and the weaknesses which contributed to his downfall in Montreal. An attempt will be made to shed light on what sort of a person Gray was and to reach a conclusion about what he achieved and what he should be remembered for.

Gray's career before the Great War-one of Aberdeen's most distinguished surgeons

Several papers in the medical literature confirm that Gray was one of Aberdeen's most distinguished surgeons who made many important contributions to surgery, including the introduction of aseptic surgery to Aberdeen. He was an extremely hard taskmaster and not an easy man to work for, but his house surgical posts were very popular and much sought after, because young doctors trained by Gray were given confidence and standing that boded well for future success. At the same time, many house surgeons must have found Gray to be a frightening figure, as he gazed menacingly at them over his spectacles from the other side of the operating table if they had failed in any part of their duty. On the other hand, if they had displayed full commitment to looking after the patients under their care, then Gray encouraged and supported them. He always put his patients first and his dedication to them was of paramount importance. He expected everyone in his team to follow his example.

There is evidence that he was not a good formal lecturer and had a tendency to become tongue tied in front of a large audience. While this failing was acknowledged and accepted in his role as a 'hands on' clinician in Aberdeen, it was perceived to be a serious weakness when he was subsequently being considered for the position of Professor of Surgery at McGill University in Montreal. If Gray had lived out his time as a consultant surgeon at Aberdeen Royal Infirmary, he would have had a notable and very distinguished career, but with nothing particular to set him apart from others before and since who have held such a position.

Gray's career during the Great War – the best war surgeon in the British Army

It has been clearly demonstrated from the literature that Gray made many very important contributions to war surgery. There is also absolutely no doubt that he was greatly admired by the young surgeons working under his direction and instruction, both at base hospitals in Rouen and in the casualty clearing stations of the Third Army. He was very supportive of them, led by example and did not spare himself. Gray spent many hours working with young surgeons in operating theatres dealing with the most appalling wounds. His constant presence and support, helping them to perform unfamiliar procedures, must have been very reassuring to his less experienced younger colleagues. In return, Gray acknowledged their energy, enthusiasm and ability. He said:

> This is a young man's war, in surgery as well as in purely military matters. The progress of events demands that younger men should have every chance in a sphere of action where mental and bodily activity count for so much.[1]

---

1 Gray, H.M.W., *The Early Treatment of War Wounds*, London: Henry Frowde and Hodder & Stoughton, 1919, p. x.

When he was Consulting Surgeon to the British Third Army in 1917 with overall responsibility for the provision of surgical services, he sometimes felt ill at ease during lulls in the fighting, because he had to delegate responsibility to others and let them get on with the routine work. On 13 March 1917 he wrote to Eva:

> In my job, I have to let other people do the work, and you can imagine how often my fingers itch to be doing things myself. Only in times of really big pushes do I take my coat off for long spells.

These are without doubt the words of a 'hands on' surgeon, accustomed to doing everything himself and having to stand back to allow younger surgeons under his supervision to get on with much of the operating. Gray would have had the additional stress of being called upon to help with the most difficult cases which others were unable to perform without his assistance. In this he excelled, helping them and encouraging them through these procedures. When there was a 'push' on, during which time huge numbers of casualties were admitted, it was all hands on deck and Gray would have been in the thick of things. When he wrote the above words to Eva on 13 March, the opening of the Battle of Arras was less than four weeks away and preparations being made by the medical services were well advanced. In the same letter to Eva he said:

> We are all very busy preparing and I hope the preparations will result in proportionately as great results as have evolved in the part of the world where your great man is. Then Germany will get wakened up a bit. You must have had a dreadfully anxious time about Ivanhoe. Twice wounded. Thank God both times reported slightly. I hope his shell shock was not severe. I can imagine what a tower of strength he is in his regiment and what a loss to them his being away, even for a short time, must be. I hope he was fit enough to take part in the capture of Baghdad which was reported yesterday.[2]

---

2 The reader will remember that Ivanhoe was fighting in Mesopotamia, where their brother John had been killed the year before.

An appraisal of Gray's surgical career

He went on to say:

> I don't think I was made for a diplomat. I prefer to 'gang my ain gait' in my own small sphere and there is so much diplomacy required. My inclinations are always to say straight out about how I feel about a thing, but in this exalted position that doesn't do.

This statement is most revealing, because Gray most certainly was not a diplomat and he usually said exactly what he felt, which of course was why he made so many enemies amongst his senior colleagues both during and after the war. As if to illustrate his outspokenness, he immediately launched into an account of his views on the rather regrettable absence of any American intervention in the war up to that time.

> What do you people think of America? Much very self-righteous talk and much self-congratulation of their diplomacy – but I cannot 'stomach' them at all. I feel they should have been in at the beginning just as much as we both being signatories to the Hague Convention. Almighty dollar! Very nice to have been able to carry out the scriptural injunction of turning the other cheek. They have not any more cheeks to turn now! I wonder if even yet they will come in.[3]

Gray's surgical skills were widely acknowledged and documented by colleagues in Great Britain, Australia and New Zealand and his book, *The Early Treatment of War Wounds*, written for young medical officers working in casualty clearing stations for the first time, epitomised the advancing knowledge of the period. References written at a later date by his peers at the request of Sir Arthur Currie when the latter was making preliminary inquiries into Gray's suitability for the Professorship of Surgery at McGill University, confirm that he was one of the very best surgeons to work in France during the war. One referee declared

---

3 America declared war on Germany in April 1917 after the sinking of American merchantmen and loss of American sailors' lives after Germany had re-introduced unrestricted submarine warfare.

him to be the best consulting surgeon in the British Army. This is an outstanding achievement which merits full recognition and he certainly deserves to be remembered for his ground breaking work which saved thousands of lives and which is as relevant to war surgery today as it was one hundred years ago. It is truly fitting that Gray was awarded a Knighthood and an Honorary Doctorate in Law from the University of Aberdeen for his outstanding services to war surgery.

Those same references reveal, however, that while Gray was considered to be one of the best surgeons, he experienced great difficulty getting on with consultant colleagues. He certainly crossed swords with Sir Anthony Bowlby, who was the epitome of an establishment figure. Bowlby served in France as Consulting Surgeon to the Forces, with the rank of Major-General, Army Medical Services and towards the end of the war became Adviser on Surgery for the whole of the British area, both at the Front and at the Base. In 1920, he became President of the Royal College of Surgeons of England, a position he held for three years. There were two occasions, fully documented earlier, when Gray clashed with Bowlby, one concerning Bowlby's paper on wound excision and primary closure and the other on his publication dealing with the incidence of compound fractures of the femur. Gray had a quick temper, was very outspoken, and simply could not restrain himself from taking a swipe at Bowlby when given the opportunity to do so. His poor relationships with his contemporaries were in marked contrast to the very good associations he enjoyed with young surgeons working under his stewardship. The reader will remember when an unnamed Professor of Surgery from London visited Sir Arthur Currie in Montreal in 1923, he said:

> They wouldn't raise any flags for Gray in London. His support in the army had come from younger men. Gray found it difficult to get on with colleagues; he was too arbitrary; too impulsive; too dictatorial.

Gray was responsible for so many advances in surgery during the war that many of his peers perhaps resented his innovative surgical methods and successes. Professional rivalry and jealousy may explain why he was often disliked by his contemporaries. Had Gray been remotely capable of diplomacy instead of acting and speaking impulsively, he may have been able to make many ground breaking surgical developments while still keeping his colleagues 'on side,' instead of making enemies of them.

Gray in the immediate aftermath of the Great War

Gray was at his very best during the war years but they had clearly taken their toll. In his correspondence with Eva in 1919, he declared that he had lost some of his drive. He confessed to feeling tired and was undecided about what to do next. He could remain in London and try to gain a foothold and become established there, or he could return to Aberdeen, but his letter revealed that he wasn't enthusiastic about going home. Nevertheless, after considerable deliberation he went back to Aberdeen Royal Infirmary, but never settled. He must have found it very difficult returning to his former way of life as though nothing had happened when in fact so many things had changed. This was a very different Henry Gray from the young and dynamic surgeon who was so clear and definite about his goals when he took up his consultant post in 1904, because he now displayed fatigue and indecisiveness. He still carried a large chip on his shoulder about London surgical establishment figures while he of course 'belonged to the ultimate division in the Sassenach classification of those north of the Tweed – the Scotsman, the damned Scotsman and the Aberdonian!' Gray clearly had an inferiority complex, which perhaps partly explained his reluctance to return to Aberdeen, considered by many at the time to be a parochial backwater. By the time he had been demobilised, Gray was nearly fifty years old and probably too old to re-adapt to peace-time surgery. It would be the careers of the younger surgeons with whom Gray had enjoyed such a good rapport that would flourish when they returned home to posts in academic units, their reputations established by wartime experience. Gray probably felt that he was 'yesterday's man' – a sentiment which ageing surgeons today can identify with! These factors combine to explain why he welcomed the chance to leave when he was offered the position of Surgeon-in-Chief at the Royal Victoria Hospital in Montreal, which normally went with the Professorship of Surgery at McGill University.

McGill University is a prestigious Canadian seat of learning and was founded by royal charter in 1821. It bears the name of James McGill, a prominent Montreal merchant from Scotland and alumnus of Glasgow University whose bequest in 1813 formed the precursory McGill College. McGill University was (and still is) home to one of the world's top medical schools and was the first in Canada. It has now been at the forefront of education and research in the health sciences for nearly two centuries and was recognised on the international scene at the time of Gray's appointment to the RVH.

The Royal Victoria Hospital was established in 1893 through the financial donations of two Scottish immigrants, the cousins Donald Alexander Smith, later 1st Lord Strathcona and George Stephen, later 1st Lord Mount Stephen. At the time of its opening in 1893, the Royal Victoria Hospital was considered to be the finest and best equipped in North America, intended to care for the sick of all nations and creeds. Lord Strathcona and Lord Mount Stephen had made their fortunes in railways and provided money for the construction of the hospital to celebrate Queen Victoria's fiftieth year on the throne. From its early days, the hospital was affiliated with McGill University and quickly acquired an international reputation for teaching, clinical care and pioneering research.

Surgeon-in-Chief Royal Victoria Hospital

This was unquestionably the most difficult phase of Gray's surgical career and was also the most controversial because it culminated in his surgical downfall and professional disgrace. The Royal Victoria Hospital was short of money, and its President, Sir Henry Vincent Meredith was keen to fill the post of Surgeon-in-Chief as quickly as possible to make the RVH financially secure. A Surgeon-in-Chief with a busy private practice would go a long way towards achieving this goal. Meredith had first approached the famous New York surgeon, Alan Whipple, asking him to recommend possible candidates for the position. Whipple made two suggestions, Wilder Penfield, a neurosurgeon and assistant director of the New York Neurological Institute and Fordyce St John, a general surgeon at Columbia's department of surgery.[4] Both men declined the offer and having failed to secure a replacement from the United States, the retiring Professor of Surgery and Surgeon-in-Chief at the RVH, Dr George Armstrong, suggested Henry Gray, whom he knew from the war, 'but not well'. So Henry Gray was approached with a definite offer without anybody apparently knowing much about him at all.

Trouble began when he was introduced to Sir Arthur Currie, Principal and Vice-chancellor of McGill University on 27 February 1923, as the prospective candidate for the position of Surgeon-in-Chief at the Royal Victoria Hospital. Gray 'lit the blue touch paper' when he enquired what his University position might be.

His appearance in Montreal precipitated a major confrontation between Currie and Meredith, because the latter had ignored normal University appointment protocol and had acted in a unilateral and dictatorial way by offering the position of Surgeon-in-Chief to Gray and then trying to pressurise Currie into appointing him Professor of Surgery. Currie was having none of it. There is strong evidence from Currie's diary that personnel at the Montreal General Hospital were of the opinion that McGill medical policy was dictated by the RVH and Currie felt that Gray's appearance would confirm their suspicions and MGH would regard the whole affair as a plot. Relations were very strained between the two hospitals on the one hand and between the hospitals and the University on the other. Matters were made worse when the Rockefeller Foundation declared its disapproval of the method of Gray's appointment and threatened to withdraw funding for a Professorship of Medicine unless the

---

4   Hanaway, J., Cruess, R., Darragh, J., *McGill Medicine, Volume 2, 1885–1936*. Montreal: McGill-Queen's University Press, 2006, p. 113.

University asserted its policy for appointments and could demonstrate that it would not be dictated to by the hospitals. The scene was set. The hospital and University establishments in Montreal with their inter-departmental in-fighting and suspicions would soon be confronted by an outspoken surgeon from Aberdeen with a track record for making enemies amongst his peers. Things were not looking good.

McGill graduates must have wondered why on earth no McGill trained surgeon was considered suitable for the position of Surgeon-in-Chief at the RVH. They must have resented a surgeon from the 'Old Country' who was unknown to them being approached. It would have been surprising if they had not regarded Gray's arrival with hostility and outrage. There is no doubt that attitudes of young Canadians were changing towards Britain in the wake of the Great War when more than 60,000 Canadian soldiers had been killed in action on the Western Front. The Canadian Corps comprising four divisions had achieved a first-class reputation as one of the most effective fighting formations. Much of this reputation was due to General Sir Arthur Currie who had commanded them very successfully during the last eighteen months of the war. Thanks partly to Currie, the Canadians had attained a significant degree of autonomy and were not meekly subservient to the whims of the British High Command. This resulted from their experience on the Somme in 1916. Following this battle of attrition, the Canadians refused to fight under General Sir Hubert Gough, Commander of the British Reserve Army, ever again.[5] The experience of Canadians, Australians and men from New Zealand during the Great War

---

5 The Reserve Army, renamed the Fifth Army in late 1916, fought on the Somme alongside the Fourth Army. Its commander, General Sir Hubert Gough was a controversial figure. A favourite of Commander-in-Chief, Sir Douglas Haig, Gough had a tendency to act impulsively and rush into things without making full preparations. As a result, many lives were lost unnecessarily. The Canadians felt particularly strongly after sustaining heavy casualties at Regina Trench in October and November 1916, which they were ordered to attack time and time again for no particularly good reason.

accelerated the transformation of the British Empire into the British Commonwealth and most Canadians emerged from the conflict with a strong feeling of identity and self belief. It was against this background that Henry Gray appeared in Montreal.

Gray accepted the offer of Surgeon-in-Chief at the RVH despite receiving clear verbal and written warnings from Sir Arthur Currie that there was no guarantee of any academic position with the University. Gray responded by saying he was well aware that the post at the RVH did not imply headship of the University but that anyone holding the position of Surgeon-in-Chief would have much to do with the teaching of students, implying that with or without a University appointment he would be able to exercise control over teaching, which must have caused Currie considerable consternation. Following the Rockefeller Foundation's ultimatum, Currie asked Sir Edward Beattie, Chancellor of McGill University, who was visiting Britain, to contact Gray and try to persuade him to send a written statement saying that he was not expecting a full professorship. Currie hoped that if Gray agreed, the situation would be defused. Gray gave no such undertaking and must surely have realised that there was going to be trouble ahead but decided to go to Montreal anyway. A change, regardless of its serious possible implications, was better than staying put.

Henry Gray's candidacy for the Chair of Surgery at McGill
Henry Gray was not a good candidate for the Chair of Surgery at McGill. He was fifty-three years old when he was appointed to the position of Surgeon-in-Chief to the RVH. He was a clinician of enormous practical experience who had been a 'hands-on' surgeon all his life, but he was certainly not an academic and was not a natural teacher. While he had the reputation for being a very good ward teacher with small groups of students (in Aberdeen at least), it was generally acknowledged that he became tongue tied in front of a larger audience. The Chair of Surgery at McGill would have been far better suited to a younger man from a teaching and research

background. Given the political crisis created by his appointment, Gray would have had to have been an absolutely outstanding candidate for the Chair of Surgery to carry the day. It was scarcely Gray's fault, however, that he was not.

When a further attempt was made to offer Gray a clinical associate professorship as a way of getting Currie and the University off the hook as far as the funding issues with the Rockefeller Foundation were concerned, it failed. While it might have been a way to resolve a difficult issue it would have required considerable tact and diplomacy which Gray did not possess in large quantities. Gray (as Surgeon-in-Chief at the RVH) would have had to work in harmony with Edward Archibald (his junior at RVH), the Professor of Surgery, to coordinate student teaching and to form a good working relationship. When Dr Charles Martin, the Dean of the Faculty of Medicine, wrote to Gray on 12 September 1923 offering him an associate professorship, he didn't exactly make the invitation a whole hearted one. He explained that a full professorship was not possible, since such an appointment would endanger the future of McGill Medical School. The acceptance of an associate professorship, however, would go a long way towards restoring harmony. Martin went on to say that should Gray refuse the offer, then it would be greatly disadvantageous. He hoped Gray would comply to help all concerned out of a very serious dilemma. To be more accurate, it would help the University out of a very awkward situation caused by its confrontation with Sir Henry Vincent Meredith and by its fundamentally poor professional relationships with personnel at the Montreal hospitals.

It is little wonder that Gray refused the offer. Instead, he declared that he was willing to give clinical instruction to the best of his ability, should it be desired, without any academic title and would further McGill's interests from an independent position. Gray ended by asking Martin if he would send him the teaching programme for the following year for his approval, a request which must have alarmed Martin, since Gray was throwing down the gauntlet. Currie was furious but he had no option but to comply, otherwise Gray theoretically would have been able to prevent student access to patients in the surgical wards of the RVH. This unsatisfactory state of affairs led to a marked deterioration in relations between Currie and Gray, who also experienced hostility from many medical staff at the RVH and had become increasingly beleaguered.

Gray is perceived as the embodiment of all things bad

Gray became the focal point of ill feeling, as though it was he who had been responsible for what had happened. If it hadn't been for Gray, there would have been no crisis and the Rockefeller Foundation would not be threatening to withdraw from negotiations for the funding of a Chair in Medicine. Eighty years after these events took place Gray was described in *McGill Medicine* Volume 2 as an outspoken general surgeon from Aberdeen who was an insensitive man who did not care for McGill tradition. In the same work he is referred to as an untried, questionably competent Scottish surgeon who had not impressed his peers. In *The Principal and the Dean*,[6] published in 2003 in The Canadian Bulletin of Medical History, the authors went so far as to say that Gray had been 'knighted during World War I for surgical contributions of a questionable nature.' Their use of the words 'questionable nature' create doubt in the reader's mind about the authenticity of the award, diminishing its significance and helping to cast doubt on Gray's character. It is noteworthy that one of the co-authors of *The Principal and the Dean* subsequently became a co-author of *McGill Medicine,* Volume 2, published in 2006, where the words 'questionable nature' were dropped from the description of Gray's knighthood. Perhaps it was felt that a derogatory remark without factual basis had been made and was therefore omitted. The reason for Gray's knighthood must have been known perfectly well

---

6   Entin, M.A., Hanaway, J., Nimeh, T., 'The Principal and the Dean'. Artefacts and Archives/Archives et artefacts de la pratique medicale". *Canadian Bulletin Medical History,* 2003; 20(1): p. 161.

in Montreal at the time. After all, Francis Alexander Scrimger VC had attended the dinner held in London in 1919 to celebrate Gray's major contributions to war surgery before returning to Montreal. Perhaps Gray's wartime achievements were ignored and 'swept under the carpet' since the overriding policy in Montreal was to condemn Gray. His notable wartime surgical achievements would have been decidedly inconvenient under the circumstances. In Currie's correspondence, he described Gray as one who was possessed of a cunning cleverness who could turn everything round to his advantage. He was forcing himself on McGill to grab the Chair of Surgery. Of course this was not true. It was Meredith who was attempting to force Currie's hand by having Gray appointed to the Professorship of Surgery. These attacks on Gray's character certainly brought him under close scrutiny, rather than focussing on Sir Henry Vincent Meredith where such attention would have been justifiably directed.

The role of Sir Henry Vincent Meredith

Meredith must bear responsibility for most of what went wrong. When his initial attempt to appoint an American surgeon to the position of Surgeon-in-Chief failed, Meredith was thrown into a panic since he had to keep the hospital full of paying patients to solve underlying financial difficulties. He turned to Gray at the suggestion of Dr Armstrong, the retiring Surgeon-in-Chief at the RVH. Why on earth Armstrong should have had so much say in the appointment of his successor is hard to fathom, but leaving that aside his reason for suggesting him can only be because Armstrong knew of Gray's outstanding war service. The sudden appearance of Gray, whom Meredith produced rather like a rabbit out of a hat, must have angered both hospital and University personnel. Not only did Meredith try unsuccessfully to force Gray onto the University, he installed him as Surgeon-in-Chief at the RVH, imposing a clinician from the 'Old Country,' upon McGill-trained Canadian surgeons with inevitable consequences. Meredith had appointed Gray without any consultation with his board members and then bullied them into ratifying the appointment.

Gray's removal

In *McGill Medicine*, Volume 2, the authors explain in a dispassionate way how three steps were taken to deal with Gray and effectively remove him from office. The goal was to humiliate Gray during each step and this was successfully achieved.[7] They then go on to say that Gray wrote a long rambling paranoid letter in which he said that his programmes were being interfered with and that there was a plot against him. The definition of paranoia in the Oxford English Dictionary is a mental condition characterised by delusions of persecution or an unjustified suspicion and mistrust of others. From the evidence available in McGill Medicine, the three steps which were taken to remove Gray lead to the inevitable conclusion that Gray's feelings of persecution were real and were justified.

One of the criticisms levelled against the McGill establishment in the wake of Henry Gray`s removal was that the University had acted in an anti-British fashion by bringing about Gray's virtual dismissal. In fact, McGill University still had very strong ties to Britain, exemplified by a letter written in 1926 by Sir Arthur Currie who indicated that out of six new appointments that year, four were from the 'Old Country,' one was from Canada and the other from the United States. Gray's removal, said Currie, was the direct result of the method employed by Meredith to appoint Gray to the position of Surgeon-in-Chief. While this was perhaps a fair representation of Currie's position, it would have been surprising if Gray's appointment had not generated considerable anti-British feeling amongst many University and hospital personnel. The persistent and strenuous efforts which were made to deny that anti-British sentiments contributed to Gray's professional destruction tend to confirm the presence of such feelings rather than to refute their existence.

---

7   Hanaway, J., Cruess, R., Darragh, J., *McGill Medicine, Volume 2, op.cit.*, p. 115.

Conclusion

During the Great War, Sir Henry Gray was one of the most outstanding surgeons of his era and his career in France was a great success. He did tremendous work which was recognised as far afield as Australia and New Zealand, although not, it would seem, in Montreal, where his career was a terrible failure. The fundamental causes of this state of affairs on the 'Montreal side' were Meredith`s unilateral appointment of Gray to the position of Surgeon-in-Chief to the Royal Victoria Hospital and his attempt to force Gray onto the University as its Professor of Surgery. This was aggravated by very poor inter-departmental relationships between McGill University and the Montreal hospitals and by the Rockefeller Foundation's ultimatum. Gray's major contribution to the debacle was that he fell out with and made enemies of his colleagues which meant that working with them was very difficult, a state made impossible by the carefully orchestrated methods used to undermine him. If he had been remotely capable of getting on with his colleagues in Montreal, things might have ended differently, but Gray was confrontational and when he felt threatened he came out fighting and without doubt must have made life extremely difficult and unpleasant for his adversaries. His documented refusal to wear gloves in the operating theatre most certainly did not help his cause and one of the things that stuck in the minds of Montreal hospital personnel many years after Gray had gone was the memory of the surgeon who refused to wear gloves. Gray could easily have avoided this by following departmental policy, instead of which he dug his heels in. The 'gloves issue' is symbolic of Gray's confrontation with the Montreal hospital and University establishments. His fate had been sealed the day he first met Sir Arthur Currie. If 'The Sir Henry Gray Affair' had happened in the 21st Century, it would probably have precipitated an enquiry in the interest of transparency and accountability and would have generated a great deal of work and income for lawyers representing the various parties concerned.

As to whether his virtual dismissal was justified or not, the available evidence suggests that it was not. While of course there were faults on both sides, a surgeon of previous good standing and reputation was deliberately humiliated and hounded from office to extract McGill University from a very awkward situation. Currie successfully won the battle of who controlled University appointments but Gray became a casualty of the conflict. Gray made matters easy for his opponents because he was outspoken and did not care for McGill tradition. His outspokenness diverted attention away from Meredith, which proved to be useful, because Gray's sacrifice brought matters to a conclusion and allowed a speedy return to the status quo, albeit with a tightening-up of University appointment policy. In fact, it all turned out rather well.

Prevention is always better than cure, however, and if it had not been for Meredith's appointment of Gray in the first place and the very poor professional relationships between McGill University and the Montreal hospitals, Gray would never have been approached for the job. He would have lived out the remainder of his life in Aberdeen and become rightly remembered for his outstanding contributions to war surgery. It is sad to reflect that Sir Arthur Currie, arguably one of the most capable commanding officers on the Western Front, referred to Sir Henry Gray, arguably the best surgeon to serve his country in the British Army during the Great War, as a joker.

CHAPTER 7

Gray's closing years and death

In February 1925, when matters with McGill and the RVH were reaching a head, Gray wrote to Eva, anticipating the arrival of Katharine and Henry (Junior) from Britain for a holiday. He made a brief reference to the unpleasant situation at work by saying:

> Things are likely to improve soon I hope in the 'atmospheric way'. It has not been all beer and skittles, but I hope that trouble will be past before the advent of the family.

He went quickly on to say that he, Kate and Esther were moving from their accommodation at 62, Sherbrooke Street, West Montreal, which he described as 'behind the times', to an apartment block which would make life easier, even although the rent was 'rather staggering'.

Gray continued to consult in the Medical Arts Building after his controversial departure from the Royal Victoria Hospital. Given the events which had taken place, one possible course of action would have been to leave Montreal as soon as possible and return to Aberdeen. Had he done so, it would have focused attention on a part of his career which was a failure and was best forgotten. For that matter, there may not even have been a job available for him in Aberdeen. Gray was a proud man and must have been extremely humiliated by his experience at the RVH, but whatever feelings he had, he gritted his teeth, stayed on in Montreal and made the most of things by continuing to work in private practice.

After Gray's acrimonious association with the RVH and McGill University, he had no further correspondence with Sir Arthur Currie (at least according to the material obtained from the McGill Archives) until one day in February 1933 when he invited Currie to be his guest at the Annual Banquet of the Montreal Branch of the Royal Empire Society on that same evening. This society was established in 1868 to provide a meeting place for gentlemen connected with, or interested in, the British colonies. The Royal Empire Society, said Gray, was an opportunity for all those with a British connection to show their loyalty to the Empire in every possible way. Perhaps he was trying to build bridges, or perhaps he was being a little provocative, reminding Currie of the steps that had been taken by McGill around the time of Gray's removal to counter accusations made by sections of the press that the University had pursued an anti-British policy. Whatever the reason, Currie declined the invitation, probably for the perfectly good explanation that it was too short notice and he had another engagement.

Henry Gray died suddenly in Montreal on 6 October 1938, at the age of sixty eight. After his death, his sister Eva received letters from Kate dated 7 and 27 October 1938, from Montreal; from Henry (Junior), aged thirty-two, dated 13 October, from Huntingdonshire; and from Katharine, aged thirty-five, dated 17 October, from Birmingham. These letters recall in some detail Henry's last days and serve as a witness to the substantial expressions of grief and regret from family, friends and colleagues in Montreal and in Britain at his passing.

Quite late on Monday 6 October, Gray became ill. Katharine Gray wrote from Birmingham relaying a letter from her mother, 'Daddy was out at a dinner on the Monday night and towards the end of the evening had a bad attack of pain in his chest and came home'. According to Kate, Henry had told her he had acute indigestion, although she later commented, 'we think now that he must have known that it wasn't'. She continued, 'He got better, slept fairly well and next day carried on as usual – played golf in the afternoon and then did a small operation at the (St Mary's) Hospital'.[1] Katharine

---

1 St Mary's Hospital was founded in 1924 by Sister Helen Morrissey and Dr Donald A. Hingston. First a 45 bed institution located at Shaughnessy House (now the Canadian Centre for Architecture) in the Shaughnessy Village neighbourhood of Downtown Montreal, it moved to 3830 Lacombe Avenue in 1934, where it has 271 beds.

remarked somewhat wryly, that 'he refused to see a doctor'. At dinner he apparently looked ill again and had bad pain in his arms. He spent a wakeful night in great discomfort. The next morning Kate called for his very good friend Dr Scully, whom she described as 'a much devoted worshipper of Henry'. Greatly alarmed by his condition, Scully had him admitted to St Mary's immediately. Katharine wrote, 'His heart was very weak and his blood pressure low, but Dr Scully hoped that if he were kept absolutely quiet for 48 hours it would be all right. Members of staff at St Mary's Hospital knew him well, of course and were very fond of him. He had two night and two day nurses and everything possible was done. She continued, 'On Thursday morning he seemed better and they all hoped the worst was over, but about one o'clock he had a bad attack of coughing and the end came very quickly'. Or, as Kate noted, 'he had a bad turn, became very restless, then unconscious and died'. Neither Kate nor their youngest daughter, Esther, then thirty-three and still living with her parents in Montreal, were present, having been told that only if he had total rest would he stand a chance of pulling through. One person, who remained at the hospital for the entire time and stood guard outside his door, was Henry's secretary, Miss Pinkington, known affectionately as 'Pinkie'. Katharine wrote of her, 'Pinkie was up there most of the time too and she is almost one of the hospital staff by now'. A devoted elderly friend from Scotland, she was tantamount to a member of the family and saw to all the necessary arrangements and paperwork that Henry's death generated. After he died his body was not moved to the mortuary. It was taken home, where a funeral was held on 8 October, which Katharine described as follows:

> They brought him home next day, and it was decided, according to his wishes, to have a very quiet little service in the house, as he was to be cremated, with only a few friends who knew him well and loved him greatly, but Mother said that there was widespread disappointment for so many people wanted to honour him, and it was proposed

to give him a military funeral. They put 'no flowers' in the paper, but the house was filled with the most lovely ones from all sorts of people in Canada and at home . . . Pinkie said he was looking very peaceful and dignified. There had been telephone calls and messages and letters and callers all the time, and Mother said there were so many splendid tributes to him. It is lovely to think that even in Montreal he had so many people who loved him. She thought that if they had decided to have the service in the Cathedral it would have been filled with very genuine mourners.

Henry Junior, reflecting wistfully on his father's death in his letter to Eva wrote:

Thank you so much for your sweet and kind letter. You are such a sympathetic person and it helps so much. There are two big heart-aches. One (to be) far from Mother and Esther and Pinkie, and the other that any chance, such as it was, of renewing a companionship, which has always been too brief, is now gone. The shock is so much greater than one anticipated.

Towards the end of her letter Kate mentioned that if Henry had lived he would not have been able to live a life he would have wanted. She wrote:

Dr Scully told us that if he had lived he would have been an invalid – having to lead an inactive life with constant dread of further attack. A life he would have hated. This thought comforts us. He died as he would have liked to do, in the full tide of his work and having spent a happy summer.

Just before the end of the letter she mentioned a remark made by an old orderly from the RVH who came to pay his respects. 'He has gone to a place where he will get justice', he quipped and she closed with:

There is no doubt that a fair section of Montreal did appreciate him, but they never really knew of his outstanding skill at his job!

On hearing the news back in Aberdeen, where Gray's career had begun so promisingly forty three years before, the President of the Aberdeen Medico-Chirurgical Society, Dr Harold Edgar Smith, paid this tribute to him:

> Before beginning the business of the meeting, I should like to refer to the loss sustained by this Society by the death of one of whom it was very proud. Sir Henry Gray was for many years an Ordinary Member of this Society, and latterly was one of the distinguished Honorary Members. His big shining face, his broad chest, his upright carriage, his general air of cleanliness radiated surgery, inspiring confidence in patient and doctor alike, a confidence that was justified by a finished technique and meticulous pains. In his work and in his play, he remained to the end a lovable loon, quick to anger, but quicker to be sorry. In meetings of this Society, he was, shall I say, an indifferent speaker, but to me personally the tongue-tied hesitancy of his utterance, such was his personality, conveyed an honesty of purpose that eloquence often fails to achieve.[2]

Eva received many letters of condolence on the death of her brother. It was widely known that they had great affection for each other. She had been sorry to see him go when he moved to Montreal with Kate and the children, but she kept in touch with them while they were there. And she was in even closer touch with Katharine and Henry Junior when they decided to return home in their early twenties to work and study.

The difficulties Henry had with McGill remained a mystery and sadness to Eva until her death in 1968, but she always believed her brother to be an honorable man and a courageous one. Knowing him as she did, she simply could not believe otherwise.

---

2   Minutes of the Aberdeen Medico-Chirurgical Society, 27 October 1938

APPENDIX I

Gray's Publications

Publications before the Great War

Gray, H.M.W., A case illustrating some points in the treatment of movable kidney. Edinb. M, J.., 1904, n.s., xvi, 247–249.

— Transplantation of tendon for musculo-spiral paralysis. Lancet, Lond., 1904, i, 1419.

— A two-way peritoneal irrigator. Lancet, Lond., 1906, ii, 379.

— A cause of intestinal obstruction after enterostomy. Lancet, Lond., 1904, ii, 526.

— Sub diaphragmatic transperitoneal massage of the heart as a means of resuscitation. Lancet, Lond., 1905, ii, 506.

— Vaccine treatment in surgery. Lancet, Lond., 1906, i, 1099–1103.

— The operation of appendicostomy. Lancet, Lond., 1906, i, 596; 708.

— Vaccine treatment applied to tuberculous disease. Scot. M&S. J., Edinb., 1906, xviii, 42–50.

— Remarks on some clinical conditions.: movable kidney, permanent inguinal colostomy, psoas abscess, vaccine treatment. Scot. M&S. J., Edinb., 1906, xviii, 35–50.

— Vaccine treatment in surgery. Tr. Med-Chir. Soc. Edinb., 1906, n. s., xxv, 182–199.

— Duodenal ulcer; six cases of perforation. Scot. M. & S. J.Edinb., 1907, xx, 35–44.

— Considerations concerning the functions of the stomach and the operation of gastro-enterostomy. Lancet, Lond., 1908, i, 549–555.

— Motor functions of the stomach (A) in normal cases, (B) after gastro-enterostomy, as demonstrated by X rays. Lancet, Lond., 1908, ii, 224–228.

— Vaccine treatment in surgery. Edinb. M. J., 1908, n. s., i, 108–116.
— The treatment of burns. Med. Mag. Lond., 1909, xviii, 135–138.
— Modern operations for varicose veins. Med. Mag. Lond., 1909, xviii, 272–279.
— with Collum R W The practice of anaesthetics and general surgical technique. Edited by James Cantlie,. NY, 1909, W. Wood and Co. 396p.
— Ligature of ovarian vessels as a substitute for oophorectomy. J. Obst. & Gynec. Brit. Emp., Lond., 1909, xvi, 21–26.
— Treatment of advanced cases of acute diaphysitis. Brit. J. Child. Dis. Lond. 1909, vi, 358–363.
— Modern treatment for varicose veins. J. Roy. Army Med. Corps, Lond., 1909, ix, 223–240.
— Diagnosis and treatment of cancer of the stomach. Edinb. Med. J. 1910, n. s., iv, 319–333.
— Further remarks regarding the motor functions of the stomach. Lancet, Lond., 1910, ii, 1610–1612.
— The motor functions of the stomach. Lancet, Lond., 1910, ii, 1796.
— The after effects of gastro-enterostomy. Lancet, Lond., 1913, 718.
— The after effects of gastro-enterostomy. Brit. Med. J. Lond., 1913, i, 689.
— and Anderson W, Remarks on abnormal intra-abdominal developmental adhesions. Lancet, Lond. 1913, i, 1300; 1373.
— An improved route of approach to the gall-bladder and biliary passages (Perthe's incision). Brit. J. Surg. Lond., 1913, i, 200–202.
— Remarks on chronic iontestinal stasis. Brit. Med. J. Lond., 1914, i, 188–191.
— and Mitchell A, A series of cases of appendicitis in children. Brit. Med. J. Lond., 1914, i, 409–411.

— Cuthbert et al, Discussion on the evolution of the shockless operation (anoci association). Brit. Med. J. Lond., 1914, ii, 349–354.
— and Souper HR, Case of multiple foreign bodies in the colon; operation and recovery. Brit. J. Surg. Bristol, 1914–1915, ii, 714–717.

Publications during the Great War and its immediate aftermath

Gray, H.M.W., 'Hypertonic' treatment of wounds. Brit. Med. J. 1915, ii, 32.
— Treatment of 'gunshot wounds' of the knee joint. Brit. Med. J. Lond., 1915, ii, 41–43.
— Treatment of gunshot wounds by excision and primary suture. Brit. Med. J. Lond., 1915, ii, 317.
Birkbeck, L.H.C., Lorimer, G.N., and Gray, H.M.W., Removal of a bullet from the right ventricle of the heart under local anaesthesia. Brit. Med. J. Lond., 1915, ii, 561.
Gray, H.M.W., Treatment of gunshot wounds by excision and primary suture. J. Roy. Army Med Corps Lond., 1915, xxiv, 551–554.
— General treatment of infected gunshot wounds from a clinical point of view. Brit. Med. J. Lond.,1916, i, 1–7.
— Observations on gunshot wounds of the head. Brit. Med. J. Lond., 1916, i, 261–265.
— Early treatment of gunshot injuries of the spinal cord. Brit. Med. J. Lond., 1917, ii, 44.
— Early treatment of gunshot wounds of the knee joint. Brit Med. J. Lond., 1917, ii, 278–280.
— The use of liquid paraffin in the treatment of war wounds. Brit. Med. J. Lond., 1917, ii, 509.
— Notes in connection with the above articles on surgery of the chest. Brit. Med. J. Lond., 1917, ii, 580.

— Surgical treatment of men at advanced units. N. York MJ, 1917, cvi, 1013–1021.
— Treatment of war wounds of joints at advanced units. N. York Med. J. 1918, cvii, 551–555.
— Treatment of war wounds of the brain at casualty clearing stations. N. York Med. J. 1918, cvii, 407; 457.
— Surgical work at a casualty clearing station or evacuation hospital; a general outline of work during severe fighting. N. York Med. J. 1918, cvii, 264–266.
— Primary suture of war wounds. Brit. Med. J. Lond., 1918, i, 467.
— Principles of treatment of gunshot wounds at casualty clearing stations. N. York Med. J. 1918, cvii, 696; 745.
— Treatment of compound fractures of the femur at casualty clearing stations. N. York Med. J. 1918, cvii, 1181–1184.
— Surgical treatment of penetrating wounds of the thorax. N. York Med. J., 1918, cvii, 1078–1080.
— An essential principle in the treatment of gas gangrene. Brit. Med. J. Lond., 1918, ii, 369.
— The early treatment of war wounds, NY, 1919, Oxford Univ., 305 p.
— Application of the professional lessons of war to civil work. Brit. Med. J. Lond., 1921, i, 109–114.

Publications after the Great War

Gray, H.M.W., An address on the application of the professional lessons of the war to civil work. British Medical Journal, Jan. 22, 1921 pp. 109–114.
— Whiteheads operation for haemorrhoids. Brit. Med. J. Lond., 1921, 593–598.
— The prevention of deformities. Orthop. Surg. (Jones) Lond., 1921, ii, 28–37.
— Remarks on bone grafting as an aid in treatment of tuberculous spinal caries. Brit. Med. J. Lond., 1922, ii, 73–76, 1 pl.

Gray, Sir H.M.W., The effects of stagnation the ascending colon. Canad. M. Ass. J. Toronto, 1924, xiv, 93–100.

— The operation of caeco-colo-plico-pexy. Canad. M. Ass. J. Toronto, 1924, xiv, 290–292.

— Some problems of drainage. Surg., Gynec. & Obst., Chicago, 1924, xxxix, 221–228.

— Memorandum on clinical tours for medical practitioners. Post-Grad. M. J. 3: 123–125, April 28.

— Pseudo-appendicitis, Journal-Lancet 48: 487–498, Nov. 1, 28.

Gray, Henry McIlree Williamson, 1870–1938. Brit. Med. J. 2: 814–815, Oct 15, '38; Lancet 2: 920, Oct. 15 '38.

Bibliography

Books

Adam, A.J. Hutchison, *The Heritage of the Med-Chi, Aberdeen Medico-Chirurgical Society*. 2007.

Butler, A.G., *Official History of the Australian Army Medical Services, 1914–1918 Volume II – The Western Front*. Canberra: Australian War Memorial, 1940.

Cantlie, N., *A History of the Army Medical Department*, *Volume 2*. Edinburgh: Churchill Livingston, 1974.

Carberry, A.D., *The New Zealand Medical Services in the Great War*. Auckland: Whitcombe and Tombs Ltd, 1924.

Cooter, R., *Surgery and Society in Peace and War*. Basingstoke: MacMillan Press Ltd, 1993.

Gray, H.M.W., *The Early Treatment of War Wounds*. London: Henry Frowde and Hodder & Stoughton, 1919.

Gray, H.M.W., with R.W. Collum, *The practice of anaesthetics and general surgical technique*. Edited by James Cantlie, W. Wood and Co., N.Y., 1909.

Hanaway, J., Cruess, R., Darragh, J., *McGill Medicine, Volume 2, 1885–1936*. Montreal: McGill-Queen's University Press, 2006.

Robertson, E.A., in Scotland, T., and S. Heys, *War Surgery 1914–18*. Solihull: Helion and Co., 2012.

Scotland, T., and Heys, S., *War Surgery, 1914–18*. Solihull: Helion and Company Limited, 2012.

—*Wars, Pestilence and the Surgeon's Blade*. Solihull: Helion and Co., 2013.

Watson, F., *The Life of Sir Robert Jones*. London: Hodder & Stoughton, 1934.

Journals

Birkbeck, L.H.C., Lorimer, G.N., Gray, H.M.W., Removal of a Bullet from the Right Ventricle of the Heart under Local Anaesthesia. *British Medical Journal* 1915; 2: pp. 561–562.

Bowlby, A., Primary suture of wounds at the front in France. *British Medical Journal* March 23, 1918, pp. 333–337.

— The Mortality of Cases of Fractured Femur. *British Medical Journal* 1919; 1:p. 112.

Colonel H.M.W. Gray, *British Medical Journal*, 19 April, 1919; p. 503.

Correspondence; Resignation of Sir Henry Gray; *Canadian Medical Association Journal*, November 1925; 15(11): p.1163.

Entin, M.A., Hanaway, J., Nimeh, T., 'The Principal and the Dean'. Artefacts and Archives/Archives et artefacts de la pratique medicale'. *Canadian Bulletin Medical History.* 2003; 20(1): p. 161.

Gray, H.M.W., 'An address on the application of the professional lessons of the war to civil work.' *British Medical Journal*, 22 Jan. 1921; pp. 109–114.

— An essential principle in the treatment of gas gangrene. *British Medical Journal* 1918; 1: p. 369.

— Correspondence; Primary suture of war wounds. *British Medical Journal* April 20, 1918, p. 467.

— Early Treatment of Gunshot Injuries of the Spinal Cord. *British Medical Journal* 1917; 2: pp. 44–45.

— General Treatment of Infected Gunshot Wounds. *British Medical Journal* 1915; 2: pp.41–43.

— Gunshot Wounds of the Head. *British Medical Journal* 1916; 1: pp. 261–265.

— Gunshot wounds of the knee joint. *British Medical Journal*; 1917; 2: pp. 278–280.

— The Mortality of Cases of Fractured Femur. *British Medical Journal* 1919; 1: p. 142.

— The treatment of gunshot wounds by excision and primary suture. *Journal Royal Army Medical Corps* June 1915, pp. 551–4.
— Treatment of Gunshot wounds by excision and primary suture. *British Medical Journal* 1915; 2: p. 317.
— Treatment of Gunshot wounds of the knee Joint. *British Medical Journal*; 1915; 2: pp. 41–43.

http://www.ehow.com/about_6572251_history-surgical-gloves.html

Lister, J., 'On the antiseptic principle in the practice of surgery.' *British Medical Journal*, 1867; 2: pp. 246–248.
Minutes of the Aberdeen Medico-Chirurgical Society, 27 October 1938
Mulligan, E.T.C., The early treatment of projectile wounds by excision of the damaged tissue. *British Medical Journal* 1915; 1: p. 1081.
Obituary, Sir Henry Gray, KBE, FRCS, LLD, *The Lancet*, October 15, 1938, p. 920.
Obituary, Sir Henry Gray. KBE, CB, CMG, LLD, FRCS Ed., *British Medical Journal*, October 15, 1938, p. 814.
Obituary, Sir Henry McIlree Williamson Gray, *Canadian Medical Association Journal*, Dec 1938, p. 612.
Platt, H., 'Moynihan; The Education and Training of the Surgeon. Eleventh Moynihan Lecture delivered University of Leeds 25 May 1961', *Annals of the Royal College of Surgeons of England* 1962; 30: pp. 220–228.
Porter, R.M.M., Recent Aberdeen Medical Teachers: Sir Henry Gray, KBE, CB, CMG, LLD, FRCS (Ed), *Aberdeen Postgraduate Medical Bulletin*, Oct. 1971, pp. 11–13.
Sir Henry Gray, *British Medical Journal*, 24 October, 1925; p. 770.
Sir Henry Gray, *British Medical Journal*, 3 October, 1925; p. 621.
Smith, F.K., Sir Henry Gray, KBE, CB, CMG, *The Aberdeen University Review*, 1939, Vol XXVI pp. 47–49.
The Aberdeen University Review. 1923–24; XI.

The War Medical Arrangements of the British Expeditionary Force. From a Special Correspondent in France. *British Medical Journal*, 12 June 1915.

Thomas, J. Lynn., A simple modification of the Guillotine or Flapless method of Amputation. *British Medical Journal*, 1916; 2: pp. 481–482.

University of Aberdeen, Roll of Service in the Great War 1914–1919. Edited by MD Allardyce, Aberdeen University Press. 1921.

Papers

Diary and letters of Sir Arthur Currie relating to Sir Henry Gray; Archives McGill University

Index

Aberdeen Medico-chirurgical Society, 11, 12, 13, 19, 66, 154, 165
Aberdeenshire Cricket Club, 12, 13, 77, 78
anaesthesia
  local, 65, 105, 161, 166
  nitrous oxide/oxygen, 103
  regional, 65
  spinal, 65
Army Units
  4th Australian Field Ambulance, 103
  26th Punjabis, 48
  36th Sikhs, 43, 107
  Australian Divisions, 82
  battalion, 81
  brigade, 81
  Canadian Army Medical Corps, 112, 114
  Canadian Corps, 25, 115, 146
  Canadian soldiers, 146
  Division, 81, 146
  Indian Army, 106, 108
  Reserve Army, 146
  Royal Army Medical Corps (RAMC), 12, 59, 79, 87, 96, 167
  Third Army, 23, 25, 79, 95, 103, 104, 117, 139, 140

British Empire, 147
British Commonwealth, 147

Canadian Bulletin of Medical History, 19, 149
Canadian Medical Association, 126
Canadian Medical Association Journal, 130, 131, 132, 133, 134, 166, 167
carbolic acid, 11, 58, 59, 73
clostridium perfringens, 85

Director General of Army Medical Services, 91
Director of Military Orthopaedic Surgery, 91

evacuation pathway (for wounded), 12, 80, 81

fractures (other than specifically femur) 24, 86, 91, 92, 95, 100
fracture courses, 25

gas gangrene, 23, 85, 86, 88, 95, 104, 162, 166
germ theory of disease, 58, 62
gloves, 13, 72-76, 137, 152, 167
Gray
  Aberdeen Volunteer Artillery, 65
  assistant anaesthetist, 64
  assistant surgeon, 64
  C.B. (mil), 79
  C.M.G. (mil), 79
  Col., A.M.S., 79
  death, 7, 18, 154, 155, 156, 157, 158

Fellow of the Royal College of Surgeons of Edinburgh, 64
funeral, 156, 157,
general surgeon, 65, 149,
Honorary Degree, 81
Honorary Doctorate in Law, 142
Hospitality, 76
house surgeon, 57, 59, 60
K.B.E. (mil), 79
Knighthood, 142, 149
Lecturer, 66, 69, 130, 132, 139
Major, R.A.M.C.(T), 79
outstanding surgeon, 26, 138
references, 60, 61, 62, 117, 141, 142
Sir Henry Gray Affair, 19, 26, 136, 152
Surgeon-in-Chief, 18, 19, 25, 74, 114–121, 125-132, 137, 144–148, 150, 151, 152
teacher, 56, 66, 68, 120, 127, 137, 147, 167
typhoid fever, 65
war surgeon, 115, 139
war surgery, 20, 24, 26, 91, 101, 105, 106, 111, 139, 142, 150, 153, 165

Gray's Family members
A.R. Gray (Gray's father), 27–32, 34–36, 38–41
Adam (Gray's brother) 27, 33, 42
Adam (Gray's grandfather) 27
Aleck (Gray's brother) 27, 31, 40, 41, 43, 44, 50, 107
Alice (Gray's sister) 27, 32, 41
Barbara Begg Gray (Gray's sister) 27, 40, 41
Barbara Constance Stewart (Gray's niece) 40
Barbara Gray Ivens (Gray's niece) 48, 49, 50, 51, 109
Barbara Shand Anderson Gray (Gray's mother) 27, 29, 30, 31, 34, 41, 47
Elspet (Gray's aunt), 27
Ernest Simson (Eva's fiancée), 45
Esther (Gray's daughter) 45, 46, 47, 51, 53
Eva (Gray's sister), 27, 32–35, 39–45, 47–55, 69, 83, 106, 108, 113, 140, 143, 154–158
Harold Ivens (Ivanhoe), 48, 50, 51, 54, 108, 140
Henry Robert, also Henry Junior (Gray's son), 45, 47, 51, 54, 154, 155, 157, 158
Howard Coote(Gray's brother-in-law), 40, 44,
James (Gray's uncle), 27, 31
Jane Isobel (Gray's niece; author's mother), 53
Jane Reith Gray (Gray's grandmother), 27
Janet (Gray's sister-in-law), 43, 50
Jeannie (Gray's sister), 27, 32, 40, 43, 44, 45
John (Gray's brother) , 27, 41–43, 45-47, 51, 107, 108, 109
John (Gray's nephew), 51
Katharine (family name Kang for Gray's daughter), 45, 46, 47, 51, 54, 154, 155, 156, 158
Kate (Gray's wife), 42, 44–49, 51, 54, 106, 155–158
Kemo (family name for Eva's fiancée), 45, 48
Lucy (Gray's sister-in-law), 107, 108, 109
Robert (Gray's brother), 27, 31, 32, 34, 41
Robert (Gray's uncle) 27, 28, 29, 41, 60

Index

William (Gray's brother) 27, 36, 38, 39, 41, 55
William Anderson (Gray's grandfather), 30

Hospitals
  1st Scottish General Hospital, 65
  Aberdeen Royal Infirmary, 11, 19, 23, 60, 64, 65, 67, 68, 75, 77, 113, 130, 139, 143
  Alder Hey Hospital, 91
  Castlehill Barracks Hospital, 51
  Children's Hospital (Aberdeen) 51
  Glasgow Royal Infirmary, 58
  Montreal General Hospital (MGH), 116, 119, 145
  Old Mill Hospital, 12, 93
  orthopaedic centres, 92, 94
  Red Cross Unit, Wimeraux, 79
  restorative workshop, 12, 92, 94
  Royal Victoria Hospital (RVH), 15, 18, 19, 20, 25, 26, 74, 114–116, 119, 120, 126, 128, 129, 131, 132, 144, 145, 152, 154
  Southern General Hospital, Liverpool, 72
  St Mary's Hospital, 155, 156
  Woodend Hospital, 92
Hammersmith Workshop, 92,

journals, 20, 32, 33, 42, 43, 166

letters (from Gray to Eva), 12, 33, 42, 43, 44, 46, 48, 50, 51, 53, 55, 108, 110, 113, 140, 143,

Manchester Ship Canal, 72,
McGill University
  Archives, 14, 20, 115, 117, 131, 138, 149, 154, 166
  Chair of Surgery, 20, 116, 117, 120, 124, 134, 147, 148, 150,
  Chancellor, 123, 126, 147
  Dean of the Faculty of Medicine, 121, 126, 148, 149, 166
  Electoral Board, 124
  McGill Medical School, 124, 148,
  Medical Advisory Committee, 116,
  Medical Arts Building, 128, 154,
  Medical Faculty, 126, 127,
  Principal and Vice- chancellor, 20, 25, 115, 118, 121, 122, 123, 130, 145, 149, 166
  Professor of Surgery, 18, 114, 115, 118, 119–126, 134, 136, 139, 141, 144, 145, 148, 150, 152
  Professorship of Medicine, 121, 145
  Selection Board, 116, 122
  University Clinic, 121,
media attention, 133
Medical facilities in France
  advanced dressing station (ADS), 81, 82
  base hospitals, 23, 24, 79, 82–86, 102, 159
  casualty clearing station (CCS), 24, 82, 83, 86, 87, 96-98, 101–103, 139, 141, 162
  clearing hospitals, 82
  field ambulance, 23, 81, 83
  field ambulance resuscitation teams, 82, 104
  general hospitals, 92
  hospital train, 82
  main dressing station (MDS), 81, 82
  motor ambulance wagons, 82, 101
  nursing sisters, 82

171

regimental aid post, 81–84
regimental medical officer, 81
regimental stretcher bearers, 81
resuscitation teams, 82, 104
Merchiston Castle School, 11, 13, 36, 38, 56
Merchistonian, 13, 37, 45
Moynihan Provincial Surgical Club, 69, 70, 72, 91

Nellfield Cemetery, 41
neuritis, 53

orthopaedic centres, 92, 94

People
  Adami, G, 119
  Archibald, EW, 118, 122, 124, 127, 128, 130, 134, 136, 137, 148
  Armstrong, G, 114, 115, 116, 119, 122, 124, 145, 150
  Bainbridge, FA, 102
  Barker, H, 65
  Bayliss, WM, 102
  Beatty, E, 123, 126
  Bergmann, E, 63, 76
  Birks, H, 133, 134
  Bowlby, A, 89, 90, 97–99, 142, 166
  Cannon, WB, 102
  Carberry, AD, 25, 95, 165
  Carrel, A, 88, 89
  Christie, J, 39, 56, 77
  Coote, H, 40, 44
  Coote, C, 108
  Currie, A, 14, 15, 20, 25, 26, 115–131, 133-138, 141, 142, 145–155, 168
  Dakin, H, 88
  Dale, HH, 102
  Elliott, TR, 102
  Fraser, J, 102
  Gibson, G, 133
  Gordon, C, 129
  Gough, H, 146
  Hay, M, 61, 62
  Holmes à Court, A, 103
  Jones, R, 12, 24, 70–73, 91–94, 96, 162, 165
  Keogh, A, 91, 93
  Laidlaw, PP, 102
  Lister, A, 56
  Lister, J, 56, 58, 59, 62, 63, 167
  Lynn-Thomas, J, 106
  Makins, G, 94
  Marnoch, J, 69
  Martin, C, 121, 124–126, 137, 148
  McGill, J, 144
  Meredith, HV, 18, 19, 26, 114, 116, 117, 119–122, 124, 126, 128, 129, 132, 134–137, 144, 145, 148, 150–153
  Milligan, ETC, 17, 87, 89, 90, 112
  Mount Stephen, Lord, 144
  Moynihan, B, 11, 12, 70, 72, 73, 91, 93, 94, 167
  Ogston, A, 11, 57, 59–63, 69
  Pasteur, L, 58, 119
  Penfield, Wilder, 145
  Pierce, Dr, 121, 122
  Pinkington, Miss (Pinkie), 156, 157
  Platt, H, 70, 91, 93, 94, 167
  Richards, AN, 102
  Scrimger, FA, 112, 113, 115, 150
  Scully, Dr, 156, 157
  Sherrington, CS, 102
  Sievewright, J, 65
  Smith, DA, 144
  Smith, HE, 66, 158
  St John, F, 145

Index

Starling, EH, 102
Stephen, G, 144
Stewart, MP, 111
Strathcona, Lord, 144
Thomas, Hugh Owen, 71
Walker, K, 103, 104
Wallace, C, 102
Webster, HE, 129, 131, 132
Whipple, A, 145
Williams, B, 136
Wood, C, 135

Places

Aberdeen, 5, 12, 13, 15, 17, 18, 21, 25, 26, 27, 29, 35, 36, 39, 40–45, 48, 49, 51, 56, 57, 61–63, 68, 92, 94, 106–109, 113, 135, 138, 139, 142, 143, 146, 147, 149, 153, 154, 158
Aboyne , 54
Afghanistan, 35
America, 141, 144, 150
Amiens, 115
Arras, 140
Australia, 17, 18, 24, 86–89, 102–104, 141, 146, 152, 165
Baghdad, 140
Berlin, 63
Birmingham, 94, 155
Bonn, 63
Brighton, 36
British Columbia, 134
Canal du Nord, 115
Cape Colony, 35
Cardiff, 94, 106
Darjeeling, 107
Dundee, 113
Gézaincourt, 103, 104
Givenchy, 83
Glasgow, 94
Great Britain, 141
Hong Kong, 48
India, 28, 35, 43, 44, 46, 48, 50, 53, 54, 60, 106, 107
Kut-el-Amara, 107
Leeds, 70, 93, 94
Leipzig, 63
Liverpool, 70, 71, 91, 123
London, 13, 17, 20, 34, 41, 44, 48, 49, 63, 70, 75, 92, 93, 94, 112, 113, 115, 118, 142, 143, 150
Louvencourt, 95
Marseilles, 44, 50
Mesopotamia, 48, 52, 106–108, 140
Montreal, 14, 18–20, 25, 26, 69, 74, 114–119, 123, 124, 130, 131–139, 142, 144, 145, 150, 152–158, 165
Naini Tal, 53
New York, 121, 122, 145
New Zealand, 17, 25, 41, 42, 95, 106, 141, 146, 152, 165
Old Country, 114, 133, 135, 146, 150, 151
Old Meldrum, 27, 29
Pakistan, 35,
Paris, 50, 75, 119
Passchendaele, 115
Peshawar, 43
Poperinghe, 83
Roedeen School, 36
Rotorua, 41
Rouen, 23, 79, 83, 84, 86, 87, 106, 108, 109
Sandhurst, 43, 107
Serbia, 50
Somme, 146
Stukeley, 44, 45
Vlamertinghe, 83
Wellington, 41
Wellington, Ontario, 135

Wimeraux, 79
Ypres, 83, 112
Ypres Salient, 83

Press (newspapers), 130, 134, 135, 155

restorative workshop, 12, 92, 93
rifle splint, 12, 96, 98
Rockefeller Foundation, 121, 122, 123, 136, 145, 147, 148, 149, 152
Royal Empire Society, 155

Second Boer War, 85
Shock
  circulatory collapse, 24, 101
  haemorrhagic shock, 17, 101
  hypovolaemic shock, 96
  Medical Research Committee, 102
  primary shock, 103
  secondary shock, 103
  shock centre, 103, 104
staphylococcus, 57, 85
streptococcus, 85
Surgery
  antiseptic surgery, 11, 56, 58, 59
  aseptic surgery, 62, 63, 65, 138
  conditions requiring surgery
  compound fractures, 24, 89, 91, 95, 97, 98, 101, 102
  delayed union (fractures), 58
  femur, (fractures), 12, 17, 24, 71, 72, 89, 95–98, 101, 102, 142, 162, 166
  gunshot wounds of the head, 104, 161, 166
  gunshot wounds of the spinal cord, 104
  head injuries, 117
  heart (removal of bullet from), 105, 161
  infected gunshot wounds, 104, 161, 166
  joint surgery, 117
  mal-union (fractures), 92
  musculoskeletal wounds, 25, 71, 72
  non-union (fractures), 92
  orthopaedic wounds, 72, 91
  penetrating wounds of the knee joint, 99, 100
  prevention and treatment of gas gangrene, 104
  septic wounds of the limbs, 106
  thoracic surgery, 117
  tibia and fibula, 58

tetanus, 23
Thomas Splint, 12, 72, 96, 98, 100, 102

Universities
  Marischal College, 11, 56, 57
  Melbourne University, 87
  University College, London, 65
  University of Aberdeen, 11–13, 19, 23, 57, 60–62, 69, 79, 142, 168
  University of Berlin, 63
  University of Edinburgh, 56, 136
  University of Leeds, 70, 91, 167
  University of Liverpool, 71, 119
  University of Wurzburg, 63

Wounds (general aspects)
  Antiseptics, 11, 56, 58, 59, 62, 63, 75, 88, 89
  definitive surgery, 23, 24, 82, 85, 87, 96

Index

delayed primary closure, 88
disastrous management of wounds, 85
disinfection, 23, 74
filthy contaminated wounds, 81, 82, 85
healing by first intention, 87
inflammation, 49
primary closure, 87, 88, 100, 104, 142
pus, 23, 49
secondary suture, 88
septic wounds, 106
shattered limbs, 49
sterilisation, 63
suturing, 23, 87
wound excision, 23, 24, 86–88, 97, 98, 100, 104, 106, 112, 142
wound infections, 23, 85